"In working the emergency room, I frequently see the ravages of degenerative joint disease. Reading this book can be invaluable in helping you make the lifestyle changes which can spare you those unpleasant consequences. I highly recommend it to you."

—Ellis Whitehead, M.D.

"This nutritional manual is fascinating, exciting, instructive and complete . . . a truly wonderful, <u>much-needed book</u>!"

—Mary Ann Kibler, M.D.

If you have arthritis or know someone with arthritis, this is a <u>must-have book!</u>

—Harry A. Eidenier, Jr., Ph.D.

"I am excited about having such a useful tool to recommend to my patients. <u>Great book!</u>"

—Sistie Wilcox, MW, RNCS,
Family Nurse Practitioner, S. Carolina

"A concise outline of many factors pertaining to degenerative osteoarthritis."

—Donald H. Huldin, M.D., Lansing, Michigan

". . . well written and planned."—Dr. & Mrs. Lewis Minor, Lansing, Michigan

"Thank you again for writing a wonderful book . . . it has been a tremendous aid in helping people . . ."

—Jeffrey H. Moss, D.D.S.

"Great book!!!" —Bruce West, D.C., Carmel, CA; Editor, *Health Alert* newsletter

". . . well written. <u>Well Done!</u>" —Jerry Zuker, D.C., Zuker Chiropractic, Williamston, Michigan

". . . very informative!" —R. L. Wollenschlager, D.C., Toledo, Ohio

". . . This book answers many of the questions I have had in a manner which I understand."

—Bertie Arroyo, Layette, Colorado

"This is a wonderful book . . . I started doing the exercises shown in the book, drinking at least eight glasses of water per day . . . I am 86 years of age, healthy, active, do my housework, drive my car . . ."

—Donnie Downs, Dallas, Texas

". . . informative and fascinating." —M. F., Lansing, Michigan

". . . before starting the program you recommended my husband, Bob, was in severe pain due to spinal bone spurs, unable to walk a half block without stopping. He was resigned to the possibility of no longer playing golf. He is *now able to walk* well enough to work as a crop insurance assessor and is swinging golf clubs again. We both appreciate what your program has done for him. Thank you."
—Carol and Bob Padilla, Madera, California

Arthritis Relief!

Breakthroughs in Natural Healing

Dear Linda ~
thank you for blessing
the community with
your healing expertise and
care. Warmly,
Debbie
Wilcox
Jamesin

Deborah L. Wilcox

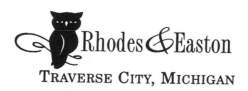

Rhodes & Easton

TRAVERSE CITY, MICHIGAN

The information contained in this book should not be misconstrued as diagnostic or curative recommendations for any disease or symptom. It is not intended to be medical advice, which should be obtained from a licensed physician.

Published by Rhodes &Easton
121 E. Front Street, 4th Floor, Traverse City, Michigan 49684

Publisher's Cataloging-in-Publication Data
Wilcox, Deborah L.
    Arthritis relief : breakthroughs in natural healing / Deborah L.
Wilcox. — Traverse City, Mich. : Rhodes and Easton, c1998
      p. ill. cm
    Includes bibliographical references and index.
    ISBN 1-890394-04-1
      1. Arthritis—Diet therapy. 2. Self-care, Health. I. Title
RC935.W55 1998   97-67979
616.722—dc21   CIP

Illustrations by Richard B. Wilcox and O'Briens Agency, Inc.

PROJECT COORDINATION BY JENKINS GROUP, INC.

01 00 99 ❖ 5 4 3 2 1

Printed in the United States of America

Breakthroughs in Natural Healing, also by Deborah L. Wilcox

Dedicated to my mentor and friend,

Harry O. Eidenier, Jr., Ph.D.

*His generous support and great wisdom
are always an inspiration.*

Contents

Introduction

Over 40 million Americans suffer from osteoarthritis, rheumatoid arthritis, or related forms of arthritis such as gout, lupus, psoriasic arthritis and lyme disease. That's one in eight people in America who have arthritis, which has increased 37 percent in just the past 10 years.

Arthritis, inflammation of the joints, is one of the oldest diseases known to man—and it is not just an "old person's" disease. There are over 100 different forms of arthritis and one variety or another can affect people in any age group, even pre-adolescents. Current date indicates that twice as many women as men have arthritis.

As people live longer and attitudes change about health and aging, we don't want to just "give in" to the symptoms of arthritis and learn to "live with" the aches, pain and stiffness.

People of all ages afflicted with arthritis or those who want to prevent arthritis are exploring natural ways to feel better. Rather than accept the idea that there is no cure for arthritis and that it is a normal part of the aging process, we are more aware of ways in which we can take action to restore our health using natural, non-invasive approaches.

Natural approaches may assist the body by supporting its normal function and balance. Unlike conventional drug therapy or surgery, which have the potential of creating side effects and masking symptoms without actually addressing the true cause of the disease, natural techniques can be complementary to other lifestyle goals and will not overburden the body with toxic chemicals or temporarily camouflage the symptoms of pain or stiffness.

The natural approaches to arthritis relief discussed in this book may be new to you; however, their efficacy has been proven by health practitioners worldwide. As you explore and practice these ideas and methods, be open to the healing forces within you. During restoration and healing, you may still have some joint pain from arthritis. Remember, the body may need weeks, months, and even years to restore and heal.

The information presented here can work in conjunction with traditional medicine as you and your physician work together. Do not hesitate to seek the advice and support of your health care professional. These natural approaches are not meant to replace the advice and wisdom of a licensed health care practitioner, your physician. Nor is the treatment meant to be misconstrued as diagnostic, curative or a replacement for necessary medication or surgery. Ideally, working with your selected health care providers and sharing this book with them can help you make informed and wise health care choices.

This book is designed to give you more choices and applications of health care beyond conventional medicine or other alternatives you may be already aware of. Don't settle for mediocre health.

Take action—apply and practice these principles early and you can prevent or slow the progression of arthritis. You'll certainly experience a sense of well-being and more energy than you thought possible. And remember, health care isn't just care given to us—the best care can be the care we give to ourselves . . . good food, nourishment, fresh air, exercise, and laughter and fun!

About the Author

Deborah L. Wilcox, Nutritionist and Lifestyle Management Consultant, is a graduate of Michigan State University. She has practiced at the Jamieson Total Health Care Center in Lansing, Michigan, since 1979 and is co-owner of the Better Health thru Nutrition practice within Dr. Thomas K. Jamieson's office. She is owner of Health & Life Dynamics™, a lifestyle management, nutrition consulting and hypnotherapy practice. She also practices in Meridian Health & Wellness Center in East Lansing, Michigan.

Deborah is a guest lecturer at Michigan State University's Osteopathic Medicine, Human Medicine, and Nursing colleges. She helped establish the Michigan State University football team's training table menu in 1981 and 1982 and lectured on nutrition at the 1984 Olympic Training Center in Colorado Springs, Colorado.

She is a master hypnotherapist, graduate, Institute of Transformational Hypnotherapy, and an Associate Instructor for the Institute of Transformational Hypnotherapy in East Lansing, Michigan.

Deborah also delivers innovative presentations, for, among others: the Capital Area American Heart Association; Lansing's WLNS (Channel 6) Guidelines to Good Health News Show; and Lansing area schools, businesses and organizations on nutrition and healthy lifestyles, using neurolinguistic programming techniques (skills to help manage behavioral changes for successful living).

Deborah is a speaker who is sought after by health care professionals on nutritional analysis of blood chemistries, symptom instruction forms, clinical nutrition and practical and effective patient counseling and nutrition management within a professional practice.

- Member—National Academy of Research Biochemists
- Member—Price-Pottenger Nutrition Foundation
- Member—National Board of Hypnotherapy and Hypnotic Anaesthesiology
- Member—Advisory Board, *Health Alert*
- Member—Capital Area American Heart Association (AHA) Board and former President, Vice President and Education Chairperson of the Capital Area AHA Board where she has received awards for volunteerism and education programs.

Publications:
Creator of "The Health Assessment Form" (a health and education symptom form used by health care professionals throughout the country).

Author of *Evaluation of the Balancing Body Chemistry Health Assessment Manual.*

Acknowledgments

Special gratitude to Hilma Wilcox, R.N.,
my loving mother, for her help in
editing the manuscript;
to my loving husband, Tom Jamieson,
for his encouragement and loving support;
to Jan Krutschewski, for her support and friendship;
to my brother, Rick, for his creative talents; to my father
and entire family, I love you all.

I also wish to thank Dee Lyons for help with typing and editing;
Sherri and Dawn Crandell for their editing skills;
Harry Knitter for his generous support; and
Jerry, Theresa, Alex, Eric, Anne and Mark,
at the Jenkins Group
for their dedication and expertise in allowing this book's
completion in a timely fashion.

*Our environment, once abundant in
mineral-rich soils, clean air and pure water,
is now no longer considered an unlimited
resource to be taken for granted.*

*Our bodies, just like the environment,
need continual nurturing,
cleansing and renewal.*

Arthritis Relief!

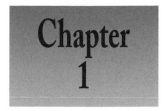
The Arthritis Family

(arth means joint; itis means inflammation)

Osteoarthritis

The most frequently encountered form of arthritis, osteoarthritis, reportedly afflicts about 16 million Americans. Osteoarthritis is more common in men in the age groups below 45 years, but tends to be more common in women in later years. Osteoarthritis involves degeneration of the cartilage of the hands, feet, knees and hips. The lumbar (lower back) and cervical (neck) areas of the spine can also be affected by osteoarthritis. Trauma and congenital problems can cause early affliction with osteoarthritis, but it is usually thought of as a disease of "wear and tear" on the joints.

Although the word arthritis means joint inflammation ("arth" = joint and "itis" = inflammation), osteoarthritis is not considered an inflammatory disease. In osteoarthritis, the joints undergo degenerative changes when the cartilage (the padding between bones) softens and erodes, causing subsequent enlargement of the affected joints. Wear and tear on the joints damages the cartilage in the joint and with damage, the cartilage releases enzymes which further deteriorate the cartilage matrix. Eventually, the cartilage thins, loses its elasticity and frays, leaving the bone without its protective cushion. Bone may then rub against bone and spurs (spinelike bone outgrowths) develop.

The usual symptoms of osteoarthritis are joint pain and stiffness, especially in the morning and in cold weather. The joints may be swollen and deformed with bone overgrowth (spurs). Proper diagnosis is made with X-rays and a complete history of symptoms.

Rheumatoid Arthritis

Rheumatoid arthritis is the second most common form of arthritis, affecting about two million Americans. It is a chronic, systemic (whole body), inflammatory disorder and is usually considered an auto-immune disease—where the whole body attacks its own tissue.

Rheumatoid arthritis usually starts with inflammation of the synovial membrane which produces the lubricant for the joints. Fluids can accumulate in the joint area as the synovial membrane becomes inflamed. Increased inflammation of the synovium eventually can destroy cartilage, ligaments and bone.

Early symptoms of rheumatoid arthritis include fatigue and weakness, generalized aches and pains, numbness and tingling in hands and feet. Swelling of the hands and feet, as well as a fever, rash and anemia can occur. In extreme cases, rheumatoid arthritis can affect the heart, lungs, nerve tissue, eyes and skin.

Rheumatoid arthritis can be one of the most painful and crippling of all forms of arthritis, and the exact cause or causes are not yet known. Proper diagnosis by a physician may include blood chemistries, a complete history and exam and X-rays.

Other Members of the Arthritis Family

There are more than 100 forms of arthritis, and the common symptoms in most types of arthritis are stiffness and pain around or in the joints of the body.

Gouty arthritis is characterized by elevated blood uric acid and swelling of the joints, particularly of the large toe, due to uric acid crystals accumulating in the tissues. Gout causes acute pain and swelling and affects one million Americans.

Medical experts may also classify chronic lyme arthritis, systemic lupus erythematosus, polymyalgia, scleroderma, ankylosis spondylitis, and inflammatory bowel disease as members of the arthritis family. However, we will limit our discussion to focus on osteoarthritis, rheumatoid arthritis and, to some degree, gouty arthritis.

It is important to note that joint pain can also be due to bursitis (inflammation of the bursa) and/or tendonitis (inflammation of the tendons), which are not actually forms of arthritis. Your physician will have different recommendations for physical therapy, exercise and treatment for each condition; therefore, proper diagnosis is essential.

"One generation's miracle may be another's scientific fact. Do not close your eyes to acts or events that are not always measurable. They happen by means of inner energy available to all of us."

—Bernie Siegel, M.D.

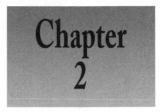

Making Sense— Arthritis & Its Causes

Arthritis, just as in any disease, does not develop overnight, but actually progresses over days, months, or years before the symptoms become noticeable. As Dr. Alan Nitler wrote in his book, *A New Breed of Doctor*, "All disease entities go through a series of degenerative stages, more or less rapidly, before the actual disease state finally appears."[1]

Over the years there has been an alarming increase in degenerative diseases, even though there have been many "life saving" medical advances. To sit back and expect medical breakthroughs and miracle cures to answer all our

Each year approximately 179,000 knee-joint-replacement operations and 125,000 hip-joint replacement operations are performed in the United States.

health care needs is dangerous, just as it has been dangerous for us to ignore our environmental pollution crisis for hundreds of years. We are finally realizing that **we must take an active role** in helping to fix the problem. Health care should incorporate a team approach where we can work with a health care professional and also *participate* in the healing and rejuvenation of our bodies.

Renowned anatomical functionalist, Pete Egoscue, who has studied anatomy for over twenty years, states, ". . . the body is not given a fixed amount of cartilage that is used up and never replaced . . . if you give it a chance the body will replace the cartilage that has scraped away. . ."[2] The essential strategy is that we must give the body a chance for healing by daily renewal of our body's needed balance of nutrients, physical activity and mental focus.

If we sit back and watch our bodies age with inactivity, processed foods and environmental contamination from neglect and waste and hope for "quick fixes," we're doomed. It would be like sitting back and waiting for a time bomb to explode.

Taking **daily** steps to heal and vitalize our body, by fueling it with nourishing foods and properly using our environment, adds up to a **big accumulation** of health benefits for our bodies as well as for our earth. This book's focus is to show you how to use your body's natural resources for correcting illness and maintaining health.

NOTES

1. Nitler, Dr. Alan H., *A New Breed of Doctor*. New York: Pyramid House, 1974.

2. Egoscue, Pete, *The Egoscue Method of Health Through Motion*. New York: Harper Collins, 1992.

"Fanaticism in nutrition can be dangerous. The science of nutrition is not an exact science, but rather an art. There are always exceptions, compromises, and special considerations. . . . there is a great physiological, biochemical, and structural difference between individuals."

—Paavo Airola, Ph.D.

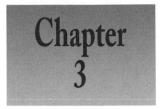
The Health Triangle

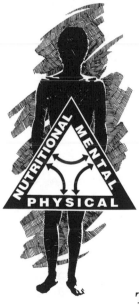

A Model to Simplify Our Health Goals

For many years, health professionals have used the health triangle, in various forms, to illustrate how the body works as a whole and **not** as a collection of separate parts. There is a functional relationship between the parts and the whole system. This is what holistic health means.

The Health Triangle

Nutritional
Food selection, digestion, assimilation, elimination, etc.

Mental and Spiritual
Emotions, attitudes, philosophy—creativity, dreams, etc.

Physical

Body alignment (posture), respiration, circulation, flexibility, tone, strength, etc.

The diagram on page 27 is an illustration of one concept of the Health Triangle.

Strive to achieve balance on all sides of the triangle. A weakness on one side will stress either one or both of the other sides of the triangle. Nurturing each side of the triangle will promote a stronger body and a stronger mind and spirit.

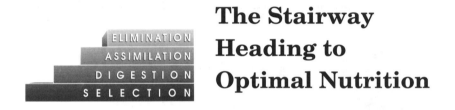

The Stairway Heading to Optimal Nutrition

The Four Steps to Good Nutrition

Remember, arthritis is not just a localized disease. It is an imbalance or disorder of the whole body. Poor nutrition can cause an imbalance in the **whole** body by failing to provide nutrients to the basic cells, organs and tissues of the body—particularly the joints, muscles, ligaments, tendons and bones, in the case of arthritis. The basic categories of nutrients our bodies need are oxygen, water, carbohydrates, fats, proteins, enzymes, vitamins, minerals and phytochemicals ("phyto" means "plant" and plants have intrinsic nutrients or chemicals continually being discovered and studied for the healing medicinal properties.)

Step 1: Selection—The First Action Step in the Principles of Nourishment Series.

1. Oxygen	4. Whole grains and beans
2. Water	5. Protein
3. Fruits and vegetables	6. Fat

1. Oxygen—the most important nutrition selection you'll make! When we increase oxygen, we can increase our energy and help our immune system. Think about this: We can live without food for more than 30 days if needed, but we cannot live without oxygen for more than several minutes. The most important "food" you can give your body is oxygen because it is vital, more than any other nutrient, to the life of **each** cell in the body.

Regular and proper breathing has a tremendous impact on your well-being and ability for self- healing.

a. Breathing is a natural part of life for us, but under stress (or with illness) we don't always breathe adequately. The best way to enhance our oxygen intake is by practicing daily deep diaphragmatic breathing exercises. Here is an example:

Breathing Exercise

	Ratio	Example
Inhale (through nose)	1 (count)	4 (counts)
Hold	4 (counts)	16 (counts)
Exhale (through mouth)	2 (counts)	8 (counts)

Repeat ten times in a row for one set. Do three sets per day (minimum).

Benefits: Improves lung capacity. Stimulates lymphatic flow. Helps energize and revitalize.

Remember: Oxygen is the #1 nutrient for the cells.

Practice the following deep diaphragmatic-breathing exercises every day. To start, as you inhale through your nose, count one. (Your abdomen should expand as your lungs expand.) Hold your breath for four counts and then exhale through your mouth for two counts. (Your abdomen should feel loose around your waistband with exhalation.) Repeat ten times for one set.

After several days or weeks, you can continue to increase your counts to accommodate the higher lung capacity you're developing, keeping the 1 to 4 to 2 ratio.

b. Activity and exercise also increase our oxygen. Stretching exercises and walking are two of the safest and best forms of activity for arthritis.

Great News!

- Studies done at Stanford University found that runners over age 50 developed fewer musculoskeletal problems than nonrunners. They also had less medication and fewer doctor's visits, weighed less and had better cardiovascular health.

- Studies have found no evidence that running increases arthritis development in uninjured knees.

In summary, the first nutrition selection we can make is **oxygen**. You can increase your oxygen intake with:

- proper posture
- deep diaphragmatic breaths
- activity and proper exercise

To optimize your energy and body chemistry, think **oxygen!**

2. Water—the second most important nutrition selection you'll make, has an incredible impact on life! Our bodies are made up of over 65% water. We cannot live without water more than about three days. It is an essential component of human fluids (such as synovial fluid in joints) and tissues (muscles, bones, ligaments). It carries nutrients, aids our digestion, lubricates joints, helps regulate our body temperature and helps with elimination.

Water helps to eliminate toxins in the body by dilution. Drinking a *minimum* of 8 cups of water daily can help reduce the pain from arthritis by helping dilute and eliminate inflammatory chemicals from the

> 70%–75% of cartilage is water!

body (that means drink at *least* 2 quarts of beverages, or 64 ounces, daily). For people with gouty arthritis, water is particularly important in helping reduce uric acid crystals, characteristic of the disease.

Tips to optimize your water intake:

a. Drink water between meals. Too many fluids with meals interfere with good digestion.

b. Eat **high-water-content foods (e.g., fresh fruits and vegetables)**.

c. Drink an eight-ounce glass of water before exercise and four to six ounces every 15 minutes or so during activity. Drink an additional eight ounces of water after exercise.

d. Stimulate your desire to drink more water by adding lime and lemon wedges, or fresh slices of other fruits, and serve in fun glasses or mugs.

e. Some health professionals recommend that their patients with gout drink only distilled water as a therapy during treatment only. Drinking distilled water (pure H_2O without the inorganic minerals and chemicals found in regular water) helps flush the kidneys and reduce uric acid levels.

f. Investigate the benefits of purified or filtered water. Chlorine and fluoride are two of the many controversial components that may be in your water and may adversely affect your health. Some authorities feel that both contribute to premature aging. A home water purification system is an ideal way to provide pure water for cooking and drinking.

Biological chemist Dr. Herbert Schwartz of Cumberland County College in Vineland, N.J. believes that chlorine causes premature aging. The chlorine in our water is not the same form of chlorine found as an organic mineral in our food. Chlorine, used as a disinfectant in water, destroys vitamins C and E due to its oxidizing effect and so contributes to cell damage.

One of the numerous research findings supporting the health risks associated with fluoride is described in the *American Journal of Physical Anthropology*.[3] Experts from dental schools, universities and health bureaus concluded that there are, among other concerns, skeletal problems and thyroid damage associated with fluoride from drinking water.

Consider reading one of the many books in your library on water quality. It may encourage you to invest in a water-treatment system for your home.

3. Raw Fruits and Vegetables—These are the most effective cleansing and healing of all foods and, ideally, these should be our first choice of foods.

In their uncooked state, fruits and vegetables have high amounts of vitamins, minerals, trace minerals, enzymes and their intrinsic factors phytochemicals—plant chemicals (known and unknown components yet to be isolated from foods) needed by every cell of the body.

The process of heating fruits and vegetables destroys many nutrients which support repair, rebuilding and cleansing of the cells and tissues.

Fruits and vegetables are easy to digest, putting less stress on the digestive organs of the body than the more concentrated animal proteins and fats. They supply quick energy and help hydrate the body with their high water content. Fruits and vegetables are some of the richest sources of anti-oxidant nutrients (minerals, vitamins, enzymes and phytochemicals) which combat tissue destruction by free radical reactions. Excess free radical reactions damage ligament, tendon and cartilage of joints.

Set a goal to eat **at least** 75% of your fruits and vegetables raw.

a. Start by eating fruits between meals as snacks or enjoy one meal a day of just fresh fruit.

b. Eat three to four fresh/raw fruits per day.

c. Have a big raw salad with **many colors** of mixed vegetables for lunch or dinner.

d. It's difficult to overeat on high fiber vegetables and fruits. They are **nutrient dense** and virtually fat-free.

e. Fresh juices made from **raw** fruits and vegetables using a juicer are concentrated sources of nutrients. Celery juice, in particular, is reputed to be beneficial for arthritis.

Fresh raw fruits and vegetables provide the most healing and cleansing effects of all foods. They are rich in enzymes (molecules of protein), necessary for chemical reactions in the body vital to life.

4. Whole Grains and Legumes (Beans)—Select whole grains such as brown rice, barley, millet, spelt, oats, wheat, rye, amaranth and quince as well as buckwheat. (Buckwheat is used as a grain, but is actually in the rhubarb family.) Try sprouted grains. Sprouting increases nutrients and digestibility of grains.

The French physician Henri LeClere (1870–1955) is considered the founder of phytotherapy. Phytotherapy is the science of using plant medicine to treat illness. Plant "medicines" are now referred to as phytochemicals (phyto meaning plant) which are nutrients continually being "discovered" as vital components or team members to synergistically support healing and repair in the body. Phytochemicals have anti-oxidant, anti-inflammatory and detoxifying benefits for the body.

Grains and beans, excellent sources of inexpensive protein and nutrients, are high in B vitamins (needed for carbohydrate, protein and fat metabolism, energy production, red blood cells and the endocrine glands).

Organically grown whole foods, rich in nutrients, help maintain better balance in body chemistry—resulting in healthier joints, bones and ligaments and less inflammation.

Quick tip to cook grains:

NOTE: To get the best nutritional value from cooked grains (such as rice, oatmeal or millet), it is best **not** to put them in boiling water. Placing uncooked grains in boiling water destroys or inactivates the phosphatase enzyme which is necessary for the release of minerals, phosphoric acid and the B vitamin, inositol.

Place the uncooked grains in the measured amount of **cold** water and stir. Cold water will activate the phosphatase enzyme to do its job of releasing the calcium-magnesium phosphates, phosphoric acid and inositol. After a brief stirring of the grains into cold water, **then** bring the mixture to a boil.

When grains are cooked in this fashion, food enzymes like phosphate can help mineral assimilation and organ function. For example:

a. phosphoric acid helps lower calcium deposits in arthritis;

b. inositol helps liver function;

c. calcium, magnesium and other minerals can be used properly in the body.

5. Protein—The protein we eat is broken down to amino acids by the body and converted into usable protein for cells, tissues, the immune system and hormones. Protein is a major building block of bone and muscle and is needed for calcium absorption in the intestinal tract.

Select most of your protein from plant sources—fruits, vegetables, whole grains and beans. If you still prefer to eat animal meat, limit portions to 4 to 6 oz. per serving—no more than three to four times per week. Ideally, select animal protein from marine fish (cod, tuna, salmon, sword fish, etc.).

The RDA (recommended dietary allowance) of protein for women is 44 grams and for men is 56 grams. Ideally, 20% to 30% of daily calories should come from protein. Excess protein (more than 35% of total daily calories) may put stress on the liver, gallbladder, kidneys and heart. Animal protein requires more work by the digestive system and produces more waste matter (uric acids, etc.) for elimination.

If this waste matter (inflammational products and toxins) over-burdens the kidneys, liver, lymph and blood system, it can aggravate arthritis. Gouty arthritis treatment is dependent on the reduction or elimination of the animal proteins (especially pork products) that cause high levels of uric acid in the blood and joints.

6. Fat—Selection of the quantity and quality is important. Most experts agree that no more than 20% to 30% of total daily calories should come from fat. Some health professionals even recommend that fat be limited to 10% to 15% of total daily calories. Presently, most Americans get 40% to 50% of their calories from fat, which the American Cancer Society and American Heart Association feel is excessive, contributing to cancer and heart disease.

Make a serious effort to reduce your total fat intake, **and** at the same time, select high quality, more nutritious fats.

    a. Flaxseed oil (also available in capsule form), the oils found in marine fish (or deep ocean/cold water fish such as cod, salmon, tuna, etc.) and raw walnuts are the richest sources of omega 3 fatty acids. This group of fats has the highest benefits for arthritis sufferers.

    b. Purchase organic unrefined "cold-pressed" liquid vegetable oils. Keep oils fresh by squeezing a capsule of liquid vitamin E into a newly opened bottle and always refrigerate. NOTE: Organic cold-pressed oils can be purchased at health food stores and food co-ops.

c. Cold-pressed, unrefined oils such as flaxseed, canola, safflower, sunflower, olive, peanut, as well as the whole foods of fish, butter, and raw nuts and seeds are rich sources of essential fatty acids. Nuts and seeds are rich in zinc, manganese and calcium.

d. **Avoid hydrogenated fats (in margarines, processed and packaged foods). Hydrogenated fats stress the liver and circulatory system because they have been refined, bleached, deodorized and synthetically saturated.**

NUT MILK

Nut milk, made from raw almonds (or any raw nuts), supplies an excellent source of essential fatty acids (high-quality fat), calcium, trace minerals and food enzymes.

Almond milk is a good substitute for pasteurized cow's milk for those people interested in avoiding cow's milk due to allergies, intolerance or other health concerns like arthritis. It is great on cereal and replaces milk in pancakes, French toast or other recipes. One-fourth (1/4) cup of almond milk supplies 53 calories, 20 mg. of calcium and 4.81 grams of fat.

Nut Milk Recipe

—1 cup of raw nuts such as almonds (blanched or un-blanched), cashews or walnuts

—blend nuts in blender to a fine meal texture.

—Add 4 cups of water slowly to nut meal.

—Option: 2 tsp. of raw honey or maple syrup blended with nut milk as a sweetener

NOTE: You will need to shake nut milk to disperse small pieces of nuts before using, or you may want to pour nut milk through a cheese cloth to strain off nut meats. Save nut meats for baking, etc.

Excellent on cereals and in shakes!! Freezes well, too!!

Our bodies need these excellent sources of high-quality fats for the skin, hair, nails and immune system. Vitamins A, E, D, K and F are all found in fresh, **non-hydrogenated** fats and whole foods containing natural fats. Use **small but sufficient amounts** in your diet to ensure good health.

In summary, to help you achieve better nutritional choices, select nutrients in this order and concentration:

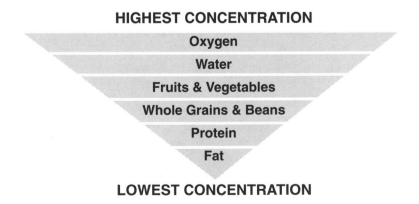

HIGHEST CONCENTRATION
Oxygen
Water
Fruits & Vegetables
Whole Grains & Beans
Protein
Fat
LOWEST CONCENTRATION

Complex Carbohydrates—50% to 60% of total daily calories

- fruits, vegetables, beans and whole grains

Protein—20% to 30% of total daily calories

- fish, seafood, eggs, poultry, meat, dairy, beans, nuts, seeds

Fat—15% to 30% of total daily calories

- oily fish, nuts, seeds, plant oils, butter

Step 2: Digestion; Step 3: Assimilation; and Step 4: Elimination

You're probably thinking, "What could food digestion, assimilation and elimination have to do with the symptoms of arthritis?" In simple terms: A lot!

One of the most antagonistic threats to the healing and rejuvenation of our body is "toxic overload" from poor digestion, poor assimilation and poor elimination. Toxic overload can be multicausal, meaning poor food selection, chemical and environmental pollution, insufficient exercise . . . and the list goes on and on.

The five steps detailed on page 40 set the stage for health by enabling the body to obtain nutrition from foods (assimilation) as well as to rid itself of toxic materials. When toxic materials are not properly eliminated from the body, they can be reabsorbed from the bowel into the blood stream where they may circulate and create inflammatory reactions, as in arthritis.

Bowel toxins can also create a pH imbalance in the bowel, making it too alkaline. When the bowel is too alkaline, harmful bacteria and guanidine (a toxic chemical of arthritis) levels increase. In addition, the assimilation and production of nutrients (like B vitamins) decrease since these are dependent, in part, on the proper acid pH and beneficial bacteria in the large intestines (bowel).

Good digestion, assimilation and elimination involve:

1. Selection of the proper quality, quantity and combination of foods, such as: (a) eating small, frequent meals; (b) eating unprocessed, whole organically grown foods with enzymes and nutrients that help digestion, including raw fruits and vegetables; and (c) avoiding excess fats and poor quality fats, refined sugars and foods high in additives and preservatives.

2. Chewing well and completely.

3. Adequate hydrochloric acid and pepsin levels in the stomach and pancreatic digestive enzyme production.

4. Good liver and gallbladder function.

5. The proper balance of intestinal flora.

Indigestion, gas, bloating, belching and heartburn can be caused from any malfunction of steps 2, 3 and 4. Incompletely digested foods (proteins putrefy and carbohydrates ferment if not digested well) create stress in the body by:

1. Upsetting the pH of the system (for example, iron and calcium both need an acid pH medium for assimilation). If your body fluids are too alkaline, calcium will deposit in the wrong places—in arthritis, the calcium precipitates out into the joints.

2. Causing diarrhea, constipation, and toxins to build up in the colon.

3. Creating inflammation from large protein molecules that are reabsorbed into the blood stream from the intestines.

We often take our digestion, assimilation and elimination for granted. Some people even believe that it is "normal" to have heartburn, indigestion and constipation and to take antacids and laxatives without discretion—and without concern for the potential side effects of these medications.

It is "common" to have symptoms of poor digestion and elimination, but it is certainly **not normal or healthy**. These symptoms, when occurring frequently, all indicate your body needs help:

1. gas, bloating, heartburn
2. diarrhea, constipation
3. foul-smelling stools
4. light-colored stools
5. irritable bowel, excess mucous in stool
6. dry, scaly skin, difficulty digesting fats

If you need to improve any one or a combination of the steps of digestion, assimilation or elimination, your health professional can help you with the correct supplements to support your needs. This support may include:

1. **Hydrochloric acid-containing tablets/capsules**
   (combined with pancreatic support in one supplement) Betaine hydrochloride (HCL), pepsin, pancreatin, ammonium chloride, glutamic acid (HCL) (stomach and pancreatic support) and B_6 as the synergist.

2. **Digestive Enzymes**
   Pancreatic enzymes, proteolytic enzymes— bromelain, lipase, cellulase, papain, amylase and protease (stomach, pancreas and intestinal support).

   > *Raw pineapple is the source of bromelain.*
   >
   > *Raw papaya is the source of papain.*

3. **Apple cider vinegar and honey taken with meals[5]**
Mix 1 cup wild honey (unprocessed) with 4 tablespoons apple cider vinegar. Take 1 tbsp. with meals. Lemon juice, apple juice or fresh pineapple juice, which are also acidic, may also help in cases of insufficient hydrochloric acid (stomach and intestinal support).

4. **Lactic acid yeast, lactobacillus acidophilus, and/or bifidobacterium**
Supportive for toxic bowel and help produce valuable digestive enzymes. Re-establish proper acid pH, beneficial bacteria and assimilation of nutrients in the intestinal tract. Make **fructo-oligosocharides** (FOS), special carbohydrates needed to add nourishment to the intestinal environment to enhance growth and balance of acidophilus and bifidus.

5. **Bile salts and betaine** for gallbladder and liver support.

6. **Special combinations of herbs and plant extracts:**

   - may contain bulk-forming agents for additional fiber to help with bowel function (for example, fenugreek, psyllium husks, flaxseed, anise, oat, beet or prune powder).

   - may contain substances specifically beneficial for healing irritated bowel tissue (for example, comfrey, okra, chlorophyll and aloe vera).

7. **Calcium bentonite (also called montmorillonite),** a therapeutic clay to aid toxin removal from the intestinal tract.

With arthritis, the essential body functions are weakened and impaired—especially the organ systems of digestion, assimilation and elimination. These impaired functions lead to inadequate assimilation of nutrients from the foods you eat. The assimilation of calcium requires an acid pH, a balance of the mineral phosphorous and essential fatty acids (vitamin F). Improper calcium utilization has long been associated with arthritis. If your system is too alkaline, the phosphorous is too low or there are too few essential fatty acids, calcium can then precipitate out of the blood and into the joints—causing osteoarthritis.

When supporting your digestive function, it is worthwhile to investigate the role that **cooked** and **pasteurized foods** play in upsetting the body chemistry. Cooking and heating foods at high temperatures (pasteurization, sterilization and frying, for example) destroys many necessary enzymes and other nutrients necessary for food digestion and assimilation. Pasteurization of milk and improper cooking of grains destroys an enzyme called phosphatase.[6] This enzyme helps release phosphoric acid which is necessary for proper calcium and iron assimilation in the body and also helps release the B vitamin, inositol.

The chemical reactions in your body are dependent on enzymes. The nutrients in your body, especially vitamins and minerals, could not work without enzymes. We derive enzymes from raw foods or foods with low heat processing from digestive juices and from metabolic processes. However, with inadequate raw foods in the diet, we are, in essence, "enzyme deficient" and this creates more body chemistry imbalance as vitamins, minerals, amino acids, carbohydrates and fats cannot be utilized correctly for—among other things—joint function and repair.

Weston Price, D.D.S., author of *Nutrition and Physical Degeneration*, gives provocative evidence about how processed, packaged, pasteurized foods contribute to degenerative diseases such as arthritis.[7] Ingestion of heated and processed foods not only upsets digestion, assimilation and elimination, but also stresses the immune system (the white blood cell count increases significantly with the amount of cooked foods in the diet), according to Paul Kouchakoff, M.D.[8]

The Organs of Digestion, Assimilation and Elimination

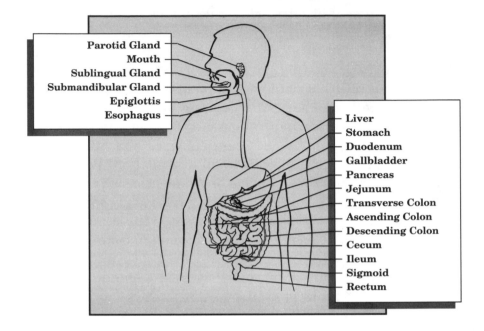

Parotid Gland
Mouth
Sublingual Gland
Submandibular Gland
Epiglottis
Esophagus

Liver
Stomach
Duodenum
Gallbladder
Pancreas
Jejunum
Transverse Colon
Ascending Colon
Descending Colon
Cecum
Ileum
Sigmoid
Rectum

A Holistic Approach to Digestion, Assimilation and Elimination Problems

Inadequate digestive enzymes and hydrochloric acid in the stomach and/or pancreas (north of the large intestine) can contribute to malnutrition, food intolerance and even constipation or diarrhea. Insufficient bile, produced in the liver and stored in the gallbladder, may contribute to improper digestion and assimilation of fat, fat-soluble vitamins, and minerals. The health of the large intestine (south of the stomach) depends also on proper bile consistency.

A holistic approach to treatment of bowel problems should emphasize selection of high-fiber raw foods, proper digestion and liver and gallbladder support where indicated. Constipation, for example, may be caused by poor food selection and digestion and cannot be corrected adequately without fixing the organ systems above the bowel first. Bowel toxins, like guanidine (a very alkaline chemical toxin), can accumulate with constipation. Guanidine will aggravate arthritic inflammation and, due to its alkalinity, will upset calcium's distribution into the proper tissues. In other words, you have to correct the problem from north to south.

"Leaky gut" or intestinal permeability can aggravate the progression of inflammatory "agents" in the body. Intestinal permeability can allow bacterial toxins, small particles of undigested food, and other toxic micro-organisms to leak or pass through the intestinal lining into the blood stream. These toxins are perceived by the body as foreign substances, thus creating an immune response and a series of immulogical responses to the body's own tissue, potentially creating an autoimmune or musculoskeletal inflammatory disease. If the intestinal wall's protective barrier is weakened further (due to an imbalance of healthy nutrients, toxins and/or constipation), more harmful bacteria are created in the intestinal tract and more inflammation of the intestinal tissue occurs.

NOTES

3. *American Journal of Physical Anthropology*, 1989. (78: 79–92).

4. Jenkins, R.T. and Rooney, P.J., et al., *British Journal of Rheumatology*, 1987. (26: 103–107).

5. Jarvis, D.C., M.D., *Arthritis and Folk Medicine*, New York: Holt, Rinehart, and Winston, 1958.

6. Douglass, William Campbell, M.D., *The Milk of Human Kindness is not Pasteurized.*

7. Price, Weston, D.D.S., *Nutrition and Physical Degeneration*, San Diego: Price-Pottenger Nutrition Federation, 1939.

8. Kouchakoff, Paul, M.D., *The Influence of Food Cooking on the Blood Formula of Man,* Institute of Clinical Chemistry, 1930.

"... the life in our bodies seems to have an incredible capacity to heal itself, if given the proper conditions ...."

—Robert Mendelsohn, M.D.

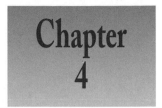

Chapter 4

Allergies & Arthritis

Food allergies, or what some allergists may categorize as food "sensitivities," may be a culprit in joint pain, especially with rheumatoid arthritis. In the *Journal of the American Medical Association* (April 9, 1992), Charles Lucas, M.D., and Lawrence Power, M.D., of the Detroit Medical Center, state that arthritis is multifactorial, but they have linked the role of food allergies with rheumatoid arthritis in their studies.

And Jonathon Wright, M.D., contends that osteoarthritis has a relationship with allergies—particularly with the nightshade family (potatoes, peppers, eggplants and tomatoes) of foods.[9] Solanine, a naturally occurring toxin in the nightshade foods, may be the contributing factor in some sensitive individuals. In solanine-sensitive individuals, solanine penetrates the immune barrier and is toxic. The nightshade foods are a source of a saponic irritant chemical that can cause red blood cell destruction. Whether or not your arthritis may be aggravated by allergies is certainly worth investigating with the help of your health professional. Theron Randolf, M.D., considered the pioneer in environmental medicine, believes in the link between arthritis and allergies,[10] and has worked with numerous arthritis patients by helping them detect and eliminate allergens from their diets. But why do foods aggravate arthritis?

One reason why foods may cause inflammation is that incomplete digestion of proteins in foods allows large molecules of protein parts to pass from the bowel through the intestinal wall into the blood stream.[11] When these large molecules, which are peptides and amino acids, are in the blood stream, the body may react to them as if they were foreign invaders and create antibody reactions—immune reactions. This is now referred to as leaky gut syndrome or intestinal permeability. This condition allows inflammatory blood cells to migrate into arthritic joints and inflammation results. In Chapter 5, we will discuss nutritional support to rejuvenate a leaky gut syndrome.

> Gluten (a protein component found in all grains except rice; corn and millet are low in gluten) can be a culprit in arthritis inflammatory reactions, according to Raymond Shatin, Alfred Hospital, Melbourne, Australia.

Detection and elimination of foods that may be creating "allergic-arthritic" reactions can be difficult, so work with a health professional experienced in this area.

Today, an elimination diet as described on page 49 is used by many people and recommended by many allergists. As you can see, it takes some detective work, devoted time, and is not 100% accurate because symptom evaluation can be so subjective. Yet, this method may uncover some food allergies that other allergy tests miss.

Elimination Diet

Here is one method of food allergy detection (often referred to as elimination diet):

1. Keep a detailed **food** and **symptom diary** for *at least* ten days.

2. Refer to this list of the 12 most common allergenic/sensitive foods:

1. cow's milk	5. corn	8. shrimp,	10. walnuts &
2. wheat	6. eggs	other shellfish	almonds
3. yeast	7. beef	9. chocolate	11. pork
4. soy			12. peanuts

3. Remember: Some potential allergens are ingredients in many foods (for example, cow's milk in baked goods and desserts; and yeast in breads and condiments.

4. Make a **list** of suspected **allergens/sensitivities**; e.g., does drinking milk cause more joint pain?

5. **Eliminate** foods you suspect are allergens for at least one week to ten days. Monitor symptoms and evaluate whether there is a reduction or elimination of joint pain or inflammation.

6. In the week to 10-day elimination period, eat turkey, brown rice, vegetables (except corn or other vegetables you are testing) and fresh fruit.

7. Your health professional may recommend that you reintroduce the foods you suspected as allergens **after 1 week to 10 days or even up to 30 days**. Reintroduce just one food at a time and only one per week. If, after reintroducing the food, your symptoms return or increase, the food is probably an allergen and should not be reintroduced again for at least nine months, if at all.

Some doctors actually recommend that only one type of fruit, one vegetable, one grain (rice is preferable) and one protein (turkey) be eaten each day *in unlimited amounts*. This is called a mono diet.

Discuss food allergy/sensitivity testing with your health professional experienced in allergy/ sensitivity programs. They may recommend a blood test called IgG4/IgE Food Allergy Screening. The test ordered by your physician, can assist in detection of food allergies.

Work with your health professional in detecting and eliminating the foods (allergens) to which you may be sensitive. Develop a good nutritional menu and work on improving your immune system and digestive system to enhance your whole body chemistry. The foods and supplements discussed in Chapter 6 are rejuvenating for the immune system and intestinal tract.

a. Increase the amounts of fresh raw food in your diet (from allowed foods).

b. Drink more water—at least 1 oz. of water for every 2 lbs. of body weight. (for example, a 120 lb. person should consume 60 ounces, or about seven 8-ounce glasses of water daily).

c. Consume small meals that will not stress the digestive system. Large meals containing processed, over-cooked foods create more work for the digestive system.

NOTES

9. Wright, Jonathon V., M.D., *Dr. Wright's Book of Nutritional Therapy*, Emmaus, PA: Rodale Press, Inc., 1979.

10. Randolf, Theron, M.D., *Clinical Ecological*, ed. L.D. Dickey. Springfield, IL: Charles C. Thomas.

11. Hemmings, W.A., "Food Allergy," *Lancet Magazine*, March 18, 1978 (p. 608).

"Nature has been making normal birds, butterflies and animals for millions of years. If wild animals can do it why can we not? Is it because they, by their instinct, select the right foods and do not meddle with nature's food by changing them?"

—Dr. Weston Price.
Nutrition and Physical Degeneration.
San Diego, Price-Pottenger
Nutritional Foundation, 1939.

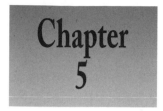

Liver, Gallbladder & Bowel Function

The liver has more functions than any other organ in the body. For example, proteins are made in the liver from amino acids derived from food digestion. Energy is stored in the form of glycogen and fat. Hormones are recycled and many vitamins and minerals are made active. The healthy liver filters toxins from the blood and transforms them to less toxic substances that can be filtered by the kidneys and excreted through the bowel. The liver is the main detoxifying organ of the body, and our modern-day life-styles and environmental pollution can put a lot of stress on this function. With unhealthy function, the liver cannot adequately detoxify.

The healthy liver filters toxins from the blood and transforms them to less toxic substances that can be filtered by the kidneys and excreted through the bowel. In arthritis, the liver is often sluggish and the entire body can become toxic—especially the bowel. Unmodified toxins can also be stored in the nervous system, brain or fat tissues.

With bowel toxicity, constipation and/or diarrhea, there may be a build-up of a chemical called guanidine. Guanidine is a very alkaline substance, and it will make the bowel (which should have an acid pH) too alkaline—thus further aggravating bowel problems. In the body's circulation, guanidine upsets the alkaline-acid balance also. When the body is too alkaline, calcium will precipitate into the wrong places, especially the joints, which then causes or aggravates arthritis.

To help support the liver and bowel function, it is important to eat a high-fiber diet, moderate in fat (using high-quality fats and avoiding hydrogenated fats is important) and rich in nutrients and enzymes. Lots of water and high-water-content foods are beneficial. In addition, you may stimulate the liver and gallbladder functions by consuming raw beets which contain an alkaloid called betaine. Betaine helps stimulate fat and cholesterol regulation and thins the bile produced in the liver. Proper bile flow is necessary since it influences assimilation of certain minerals like manganese—important in ligament and tendon support.

Beneficial for the Liver and Gallbladder:

- fresh carrot juice or beet juice

- raw fruits and vegetables

- fresh kale as well as many dark green vegetables

- alfalfa—sprouts or greens

- vitamins C, E, carotenoids, and the amino acids, taurine, L-glutamine and L-Cysteine

The following is a program to help support your liver and gallbladder.[12]

Liver-Gallbladder Cleanse

Your liver, gallbladder and colon work together to keep you healthy. When you consume too much fat, they must work harder. To encourage bowel movements, and to aid your liver and gallbladder, fresh beets are a remarkable food. Besides getting more beets into your diet, this six-week program will stimulate your gallbladder, your liver and colon:

- For one week, drink pure apple juice (organically grown and fresh-pressed is ideal). Try to drink one quart daily.

  At the same time:

- Take a teaspoon of the mixture below every hour or two during the day for three days. After the first three days, take two tablespoons of the mixture three times daily before meal for a week.

- After the initial ten days, continue taking two tablespoons of the mixture three times a day, three days a week, for a month.

Recipe:

Mix one cup of finely shredded raw beets (preferably organically grown); two tablespoons of either virgin first-pressed olive oil or raw flaxseed oil; and the juice of half a lemon. Flaxseed oil is available in health food stores. This is a powerful flush for your liver and gallbladder. It will not only help overcome the effects of the holidays (such as overdoing on rich desserts and alcohol), it will help stimulate better digestion in general, help lower blood fats (cholesterol and triglycerides) and help you regain energy.

In fresh kale and alfalfa (as well as raw sugar cane juice, raw cream and soy extracts), there is an entity which can decrease the stiffness associated with arthritis conditions. Research at the University of Oregon isolated this anti-stiffness factor, **stigmasterol**, now called the **Wulzen Factor** (named after

Dr. Wulzen, its discoverer). Stigmasterol can help improve the flexibility of joints.

Health professionals who are familiar with the Wulzen Factor can recommend a food supplement for their arthritis patients which contains the anti-stiffness factor, trace minerals, as well as other nutritional support for the liver, such as betaine, discussed earlier, and milk thistle and Ayurvedic herbs.

Milk Thistle (Silybum maranum)—an herbal supplement beneficial for supporting liver function and maintenance.

Ayurvedic Herbal Support—Ayurveda is a 5,000-year-old science of health, living and spirituality originating in India. Nutrition and herbs are foundational parts of its application.

   a. Tinospora cordifolia—may benefit immune system and support liver function.

   b. Berberis aristata—helps speed recovery and normalization of liver function with viral infections, for example.

   c. Picorrhiza Kurrua—helps to reduce inflammation due to its high flavinoid content.

These are just three of the many Ayurvedic herbs and their benefits to the liver, related to arthritis support. Consult individual product-recommended dosages. Do *not* use these herbs during pregnancy or lactation.

Liver-Bowel Clearing Using a Coffee Enema

Coffee Enema
To Support Liver Clearing

Benefits: Detoxification of liver and sigmoid area of the colon.

The sigmoid colon and liver have a circulation system in common, called the entero-hepatic circulatory system.

When brewed coffee (which contains alkaloid chemicals) enters the sigmoid colon area, the alkaloids stimulate production of the enzyme glutathione s-transferase, which affect toxins degradation and clearing in the liver to be eliminate through the urine.

Needed Supplies:
   Freshly ground coffee for brewing (not instant)—3 tablespoons
   Distilled water—2 cups.
   Coffee-brewing machine
   Urethral catheter—"16f"
   Enema bag
   Sesame or olive oil for lubricating urethral catheter

Directions:

1. Brew or perk freshly ground coffee using 3 tablespoons of ground coffee for each 2 cups of distilled water.
2. Dilute this 1 pint mixture after brewing and use as a fluid to be retained in the rectum. [If your coffee pot will only brew 1 cup, then skip step 2.] Allow fluid to warm to body temperature.
3. Lie on the floor on your left side with the left leg straight and the right leg flexed.
4. Use the "16f" urethral catheter that has been lubricated with olive or sesame oil. Gently insert the catheter after attachment to the enema bag tube and raise bag 2 1/2 to 3 feet.
5. Allow warm water to enter the rectum slowly and hold to tolerance (or approximately 15 seconds). Carefully stand up and evacuate in toilet. Repeat procedure until rectum elimination is clear or "clean."
6. Finally, start step 3 again; this time injecting coffee preparation as described above.

Please note: Lemon juice may be substituted for the brewed coffee (3 tablespoons fresh lemon juice in 2 cups distilled water).

Bowel Function

A healthy small and large intestinal tract (the small and large bowel) is vital due to its roles in:

a. providing a tissue barrier, impermeable to toxins leaking back into blood stream (toxins which would eventually tax the liver function and impose more toxins to other body cells and tissues.

b. creating and maintaining an environment of a healthy balance of micro-organisms (micro flora) and proper pH.

c. eliminating toxins with regular bowel movements.

Increased intestinal permeability of the small and large bowel (or leaky gut syndrome) is a complex set of cell tissue and chemical changes in the intestinal tract which can contribute to musculoskeletal inflammatory problems (including osteo and rheumatoid arthritis) in many individuals.[13]

The importance of healthy gatekeepers of the intestinal tract

Imagine your intestinal tract lining is like a strong fence with gates that allow entrance of your allies and guard or barrier against your enemies. The mucosal cells lining your intestinal tract act like this fence.

When the mucosal cells lining the surface of the intestinal tract are healthy and functioning well, they absorb nutrients into the body *and* also are a guard fence to keep non-nutrients and non-beneficial molecules from re-entering the body. When the mucosal cells (gastrointestinal) cells are unhealthy or not functioning well, intestinal permeability lets the guard down, compromising the immune system.[14]

Proper support for "leaky gut syndrome" that your health professional will recommend may include: (Be sure to consult your health professional. Individual needs vary.)

1. Proper identification with the use of symptom history and a Comprehensive Stool and Digestive Analysis (see Appendix I for laboratories). The Comprehensive Stool and Digestive Analysis (CSDA) is a laboratory test of 10 different criteria including: hydrochloric acid, pancreatic enzyme; bile insufficiency; parasites; candida overgrowth; potential food allergy; and intestinal motility measures.

2. Nutritional supplement support for healing and repair.

Nutrients that promote intestinal health:

- L-glutamine
- gluthathione
- quercitin and other anti-oxidants
- zinc
- folate
- pantothenic acid

See chapter 8 for more information on the benefits of these nutrients

---

3. Detoxification/clearing of intestinal tract—herbs, antioxidants, sulphur amino acids and homeopathic remedies (**avoid herbal detoxification during pregnancy and lactation**).

NOTES

12. Information used, with permission, from the *Health Alert Newsletter*, 1992, Volume 8, Issue 1, P.O. Box 22620, Carmel, CA 93922-2620. (408) 372-2103. Published by Bruce West, D.C.

13. Rooney, P.F., et. al. "A Short Review of the Relationship Between Intestinal Permeability and Inflammatory Joint Disease." *Clin and Exper Rheumatol* 1990; 75–83.

14. Smith, M.D., et. al. "Abnormal Bowel Permeability in Ankylosing Spondylitis and Rheumatoid Arthritis." *J Rheumatol* 1985; 12:299–305.

"Fewer than one-half of one percent of the planet's 250,000 species of higher plants have been exhaustively analyzed for their chemical composition and medicinal properties."

—Rosita Arvigo.
Sastun
Arvigo, Rosita. *Sastun*. Harper Collins, 1994.

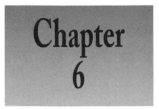

Drug Cautions

—Warning Notes Concerning Pain-control and Anti-inflammatory Drugs

One of the primary objectives of this book is to share with you information you can use to compare and evaluate what treatment programs would work best for your individual needs. You, your health care professional, and other members of your health care team can design a specialized program using the appropriate strategies in this book.

If you are currently taking, or if you are considering taking, any over-the-counter or prescription drugs as part of your program, it is important that you learn about their potential complications or side effects.

Aspirin and Non-steroidal Anti-inflammatory Drugs

The main medications used for the treatment of arthritis are non-steroidal anti-inflammatory drugs (NSAIDs). The most common NSAIDs are aspirin and Ibuprofen (Motrin, Advil, Nuprin). Many of these are now available over the counter, without a prescription.

These drugs are used to reduce pain (analgesic effect) and inflammation. The mechanism of action of NSAIDs is to suppress the formation of certain prostaglandins and related chemicals and compounds involved in the production of inflammation and pain.

NSAIDs can have potential side effects, especially when overused, that include gastric inflammation, allergic reactions, fluid retention, bleeding and bruising and, later, possible liver and kidney damage. Aspirin can increase urinary excretion of vitamin C, potentially aggravating a vitamin C deficiency.

NSAIDs can inhibit the synthesis of chondroitin sulfates and other proteoglycans. When overused, they *can inhibit cartilage repair and growth* by inhibiting collagen matrix synthesis and can actually damage the cartilage.

So let's explore the supplemental nutritional support to, first of all, reduce pain; second, to alleviate inflammation; and third, to heal and rejuvenate the joint area (cartilage, bone, tendons, ligaments, muscle). In the following chapters, you'll discover which foods, nutrient supplements and herbs act as natural pain killers (analgesics) and natural anti-inflammatory agents.

Steroid Prescriptions

In severe cases of inflammation, adrenocorticol steroids (such as Prednisone and cortisone) may be prescribed. These can reduce inflammation, but also act to support adrenal cortex insufficiency.

The potential side effects of these steroids include: water retention (edema), potassium loss, lowered muscle mass, osteoporosis, tendon rupture, impaired wound healing, vertigo, menstrual disorders, and inflammation of the pancreas.

To support the body chemistry and avoid potential side effects, as described above, consider the following:

1. Nutritional supplements with potassium, a wide spectrum trace mineral, macro-mineral and vitamin supplement designed to support the immune system.

2. Where needed, a formula to prevent osteoporosis (calcium citrate, magnesium, boron, silicon, B vitamins and vitamin K) and

3. A broad spectrum amino acid supplement to support potential wound healing and reduction of muscle mass.

These are good cautionary measures to avoid potential steroid medication side effects.

Please remember that information can fuel our education, and we must choose to use the information wisely.

NEVER discontinue any prescription medications without your doctor's supervision because it may cause dangerous effects. So consult your doctor and an appropriate and healthy method can be prescribed to "taper" you off of the medication(s), if you so desire.

"*. . . vitamins [are]* **biological complexes**, *bundles of enzymes and trace minerals, biological wheels . . . you have to have the whole complex to get vitamin* **function**."

—Dr. Bernard Jensen and Mark Anderson.
Empty Harvest.
New York, Avery Pub., 1990.

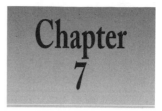

Chapter 7

Repair and Maintenance of Cartilage

The place in your body where two or more bones or cartilage comes together is called the joint. Your cartilage acts to absorb shock and reduce friction in your joints.

Cartilage is made up of three main substances:

1. water—70% to 75% of cartilage

2. collagen—15% to 20% of cartilage

3. proteoglycans—2% to 10% of cartilage

The foundation of **cartilage** is **collagen**, a protein with a helical or spiral structure that forms a fibrous network allowing resistance to tensile force (i.e., longitudinal stress). *One* of the building blocks of **collagen** is **glucosamine**, a naturally occurring amino sugar (gluco = sugar; amine = amino acid). This amino sugar, nutritionally helps support healthy joints and the body's ability to regenerate connective tissue (cartilage, ligaments, tendons) by stimulating the synthesis of collagen in joints. **Glucosamine** is also one of the compounds helpful in forming and maintaining the consistency of the lubricating fluids (synovial fluids) and tissues in and around joints and vertebral areas. **Glucosamines** also make **chondroitin sulfates** which produce **proteoglycans** in a series of steps involving nutritional cofactors.

Proteoglycans, the third component of cartilage, has a high affinity for water and together with its interaction with collagen fibrils, gives cartilage resistance to weight-bearing forces. Proteoglycan's cushioning effects are in equilibrium with the "restraining net" effect of the collagen fibers.

Chondrocytes are the cells in cartilage where the **chondroitin sulfates** are found. Chondroitin sulfates make collagen and proteoglycans. The **chondrocyte** cells receive their nourishment from a diffusion of nutrients through the cartilage matrix from a "distant" blood supply in the bone and synovial fluid. **Cartilage** does not have its own direct blood supply, so you can appreciate how important it is to have adequate circulation, mobility and nourishment to the joints.

Imagine that when there is joint damage from an injury (as in osteoarthritis) or an inflammatory disease creating edema and swelling (as in rheumatoid arthritis), there is extreme reduction of the diffusion of nutrients from the distant blood supply to the **chondrocytes** in the **cartilage**. There will also be reduced removal of cellular waste away from the **chondrocytes**. In addition, free radical damage from the injury and/or inflammatory reaction will compromise cell functions.

To enhance the supply of nutrients needed in order for **chondroitin sulfates** to produce **proteoglycans** and **collagen**, you need proper nutrition with healthy foods and supplements.

This will also help the **chondroitin sulfates** support its inhibition effects on elastase. Elastase is an enzyme released in inflammation or injury which, if left unchecked, destroys cartilage.

In the following pages, you will find convenient reference program(s) using nutritional supplemental support for arthritis, including natural anti-inflammatory agents, natural pain killers and powerful nutrients that can maintain healthy cartilage and joints, and even heal damaged cartilage and joints.

Read on to discover exciting benefits in using chondroitin sulfate, glucosamine sulfates and proteolytic enzyme supplements to heal and repair your joints.

"Enzymes are required for the proper and normal functioning of every organ system. Biochemists have described them as the 'body's life labor force' or the life energy of all organisms."

—D.A. Lopez, M.D.
R. M. Williams, M.D., Ph.D.
M. Miehlke, M.D.
Enzymes, the Fountain of Life.

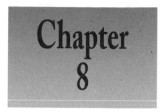

Powerful Foods & Supplements

- **Glucosamine sulfates, chondroitin sulfates and their team member nutrients that repair joints. The top ten nutrients for joint/cartilage health and healing.**

- Chlorophyll, alfalfa, brewer's yeast and kelp

- Adrenal and thyroid support

- Homeopathy

- **Natural anti-inflammatory agents, immune support and pain-control support**

Foods—unadulterated, unprocessed, organically grown foods— can really work for you. Eating healthy foods can give you more energy, help prevent disease and help heal the body.

Ideally, most of our nutrition should come from the foods we eat. However, mineral-depleted soils due to poor crop rotation, loss of valuable topsoil after flooding, over irrigation or erosion, leave our food low in nutrients, especially minerals and trace minerals. In addition, excessively cooked and processed foods, poor digestion or other health complications, medications, chemical toxins, emotional and physical stress make it challenging to get what we need from our foods.

An individualized supplementation program developed by you and your health care professional can be an asset to your body, despite what inherent factors may be limiting your nutrition. Whole food supplements are concentrates of nutrients from real food (vitamins, minerals, enzymes, amino acids, fatty acids, trace elements and phytochemicals and other intrinsic factors continually being discovered in food) to assist the body's nutrition. A proper supplement program should consider your age, life-style, medical history and symptomatic concerns (digestive distress, etc.), medications and eating habits.

The following is a list of nutrients and food sources which can be beneficial for arthritis. These are not "cures" but are concentrated food nutrition for the musculoskeletal, immune and organ systems.**

The Top Ten Nutrients For Your Joints

1. **Glucosamine Sulfates**[15]—Serve as a building block of cartilage and the glycoproteins of cell membranes. Repair and build cartilage.

Dosage: 800 to 1500 mg—3 times to 5 times daily with food.

NOTE: Glucosamine sulfate supplements *do not inhibit* elastase, the enzyme involved with inflammation, and if left unchecked can destroy cartilage. Chondroitin sulfates *do inhibit* elastase; therefore, it is recommended you use both glucosamine sulfates and chondroitin sulfates. Glucosamine sulfates and chondroitin sulfates are nontoxic and are sold as nutritional supplements.*

2. **Chondroitin Sulfates**[16] **(Ideally Purified)**—600 to 1,200 mg—3 times to 5 times daily with food

Clinical studies indicate a potent anti-inflammatory, anti-stiffness response to the purified chondroitin sulfates with osteoarthritis and rheumatoid arthritis; as well as enhanced cartilage repair due to its ability to inhibit enzymes that degrade cartilage.

Powerful advantages of glucosamine and chondroitin sulfate supplements:

1. Pain reduction (analgesic effect) and anti-inflammatory.

2. Regeneration (growth) and repair of cartilage.

3. Improvement of flexibility.

Purified chondroitin sulfates are readily absorbed (up to 90%) in the intestinal tract. The *purification of chondroitin sulfate* components from animal trachea means it is protein-free and this, along with its low molecular weight, allows for excellent absorption and distribution.

NOTE: Absorption of chondroitin sulfates from unrefined cartilage powders is extremely poor or nil. There are only a few *producers* of chondroitin sulfate supplements and even fewer that produce *purified* chondroitin sulfates from animal trachea. Shark cartilage is *not* used as a source of purified chondroitin sulfates because it *inhibits* new blood vessel growth, which would be contraindicated in cartilage regeneration.*

The Top Ten Nutrients For Your Joints (Continued)

3. **Omega 3 fatty acids**

4. **Manganese**

5. **Silicon**

6. **Copper**

7. **Zinc**

8. **Vitamin C Complex and Other Anti-Oxidants**

9. **Proteolytic Enzymes**

10. **B Complex**

Ideally combined in one or two product supplements (as whole, organic food supplements).

*When selecting nutritional supplements, look for quality and reputable companies, not necessarily cheapest brands. Some companies will manufacture supplements with fillers, binders and inferior ingredients. In addition to a company's quality reputation, you can ask the company to supply you with a "certificate of analysis" (an evaluation done by an independent laboratory) that ensures the ingredients in the supplement bottle are identical to what is listed on the label.

Please also refer to nutrient list in this chapter for more information outlining food sources, specific benefits and dosages, and Chapters 9 and 10.

Nutrient Resource List

Nutrient	Food Sources	Benefit Relative to Arthritis
Vitamin A (In plant food, carotenoids are the precursors to vitamin A. Retinols are the form of vitamin A found in animal products	Dark green and yellow vegetables and fruit, eggs, marine fish liver oil (cod, salmon, etc.)	Immune support, health of epithelial tissue (skin and mucous membranes (the important barriers against infection), gastrointestinal tract and organ linings). Development of osteoblasts (bone-building cells which lay down new bone). Important in calcium metabolism.

Therapeutic dose* (daily)—6 to 15 mg of beta-carotene or 1,000 to 25,000 units of vitamin A. Consult your health professional with vitamin A. Excess vitamin A can be toxic.

Adult RDA**—800-1000 mcg RE

1 retinol equivalent = 1 mcg retinol or 6 mcg beta-carotene

** The RDA values (recommended dietary allowances) are for adult men and women. To obtain the RDA values for children and for pregnant or lactating women, please consult: *Recommended Dietary Allowances: 10th Edition.* Copyright 1989 by the National Academy of Sciences. National Academy Press, Washington, D.C.

Nutrient	Food Sources	Benefit Relative to Arthritis
B Complex: B_1, B_2, B_3, B_4, B_5, B_6, B_{12}, B_{15}, B_{17} biotin, folic acid, inositol, choline, PABA	Whole grains, beans and peas, brewer's yeast, fruit, dark greens and seeds, potatoes, salmon, beef, pork, poultry.	Protein, fat and carbohydrate metabolism, red blood cells, nervous system, heart, endocrine glands. The B vitamins work together (or synergistically).

73

Nutrient	Food Sources	Benefit Relative to Arthritis

Notes on Specific B Vitamins:

B_3 (niacinamide) Helps joint disorders, such as stiffness with arthritis, and helps to relieve pain and swelling. B3 is required in all joint mobility.

Food sources: meats, eggs and dairy.

Therapeutic dose*—1500–000 mg/day for arthritis (under doctor's supervision)

Adult RDA**—13-20 mg

> Jonathan Wright, M.D., recommends niacinamind, 1000 mg., 3 times daily, to relieve pain and swelling in osteo and rheumatoid arthritis. *Nutritional Healing*, Vol. I, #2, 10.94.

B_5 (pantothenic acid) For adrenal support, anti-inflammatory effect and antibody protection.

Food sources—broccoli, soybeans and whole grains; lean meat, poultry, fish

Therapeutic dose*—100 mg to 1 gram for arthritis

Adult RDA**—5-10 mg

B_6 (pyridoxine) Used for relief of swollen, hard nodules on finger joints (nodes) in osteoarthritis. Helps relieve stiffness of arthritis. Relieves swelling and parasthesia (tingling in fingers and other limbs) in rheumatoid arthritis. Involved with bone metabolism and cross-linking of collagen strands which increase connective tissue strength.

Food sources: bananas, lima beans, egg yolks, meats, peanuts and whole grains.

Therapeutic dose*—50-200 mg/day for arthritis (under doctor's supervision)

Adult RDA**—1.4-2.0 mg

Nutrient	Food Sources	Benefit Relative to Arthritis
B_{12}	Dark green vegetables, fresh fruit, fish, egg yolks, milk, fermented cheeses, meats.	B_{12} and folic acid act as a team to aid in growth and formation and maturation of red blood cells. Replication of genes involving RNA and DNA.

Nutrient	Food Sources	Benefit Relative to Arthritis
Therapeutic dose*—60-100 mcg/day for arthritis (under doctor's supervision)		
Adult RDA**—2 mcg.		
Folic Acid (B_9)	Fresh fruits and vegetables, especially dark green.	(See above)
Adult RDA**—150-200 mcg.		
Folic acid, B_{12} and iron deficiencies can be associated with arthritis. Prescribed medications taken for arthritis can also create deficiencies of these nutrients.		
Vitamin C complex (bioflavinoids, hesperidin, rutin, ascorbic acid)	Raw fruits and vegetables, such as celery, grapefruit, oranges, mangos; raw potatoes, green and red peppers, buckwheat.	Adrenal and other endocrine gland support, collagen formation, bone, cartilage, capillary and blood cell wall integrity, immune support. Stimulates T and B cell transformation. Vitamin C complex helps prevent capillary walls from breaking down and causing bleeding, swelling and pain.

Vitamin C slows osteoarthritis and relieves pain. A 1996 study of 640 patients, 81 of which had osteoarthritis (OA) in the knees and 680 of the 81 with OA had OA progress. Those patients with OA who took high levels of vitamin C (1500-2000 mg per day) had reduced progression of OA and less pain.[17]

Nutrient	Food Sources	Benefit Relative to Arthritis
Therapeutic dose*—3000-5000 mg/day Adult RDA**—60 MG NOTE: Aspirin and steroid hormones tend to deplete vitamin C, so more is needed with these medications.		
Vitamin D	Eggs, butter, cod liver oil; also, through exposure to sunlight, vitamin D is made in skin tissue.	Absorption of calcium from gastrointestinal tract to blood, growth and mineralization of bone.
Therapeutic dose* (daily)—Some researchers recommend 600–1000 I.U. per day for ages 65 and above. Consult your health professional. Daily intake of 2000 I.U./day or more can be toxic Adult RDA**—200 to 400 I.U. (or 5 to 10 mcg.)		
Vitamin E	Wheat germ, butter, raw nuts and seeds, green leafy vegetables.	Cell repair, muscle tone, cardiovascular system, sex hormones. Vitamin E is unique in being able to enhance production of both antibodies and phagocytes to boost immune system and manufacture of T cells.
Therapeutic dose*—600-1000 I.U. Adult RDA**—12-15 I.U or 8 to 10 mg.		

Nutrient	Food Sources	Benefit Relative to Arthritis
Vitamin F (essential fatty acids)— linolenic, linoleic acid and arachidonic acid (also known as omega 3 and omega-6 fatty acids).	Nonhydrogenated cold-pressed vegetable oils poly-unsaturated (flax seed, black current seed, olive oil), cod liver oil and other marine fish oils (such as herring, sardines), wheat germ, raw nuts and seeds. American diets contain high amounts of omega 6 fatty acids found in vegetable oils, hydrogenated fats (margarine) and meat. Omega 3 f.a. are deficient in our diets and the best source is flaxseed oil. Fish oil supplements may contain contaminants from ocean pollution.	Mineral metabolism (calcium, iodine), skin, hair, nails. Essential fatty acids are metabolized to prostaglandins, hormone-like substances needed for immune support. Specific prostaglandins also support the reduction of inflammation and help in hormone and nervous system functions. Necessary components of cartilage, bone and all other cellular membranes. Numerous functions in bone development, structure and function.

Nutrient	Food Sources	Benefit Relative to Arthritis

Therapeutic dose*—(Consult your health professional.)—Linolenic (omega 3 fatty acids) are mainly needed. Use one to two tbsp./day of flaxseed oil or one to three capsules/day of flaxseed capsules (630 mg flaxseed oil/capsule).

Another rich source of linolenic acid is black current seed oil capsules (280 mg of oil/capsule) as gamma linolenic acid (GLA).

Flaxseed oil (an omega 3 fatty acid) is highly recommended for arthritis. In his book, **Superimmunity for Kids**, Leo Galland, M.D., illustrates how the quantity and quality of essential fatty acids is necessary for immune support. Rheumatoid arthritis, formerly rare in adolescents, is now increasing. Auto-immune and inflammatory diseases are rare in populations whose diets are high in essential fatty acids and low in saturated fats, according to Dr. Galland. Essential fatty acids (such as omega 3 fatty acids in flaxseed oil, marine fish and raw walnuts) are converted to special hormones which help reduce inflammation and support the immune system. The teammates in this conversion are vitamins A, B6, C, E and the minerals magnesium, zinc, copper and selenium. Flaxseeds have been part of the human diet for over 5,000 years and are one of the richest sources of omega 3 fatty acids.

Marine fish (cod, mackerel, salmon, etc.) contain high levels of omega 3 fatty acids. Eating 3 to 4 servings per week has been found to have anti-inflammatory effects.[18]

| **Vitamin K** | All vegetables, especially raw, green vegetables. | Blood clotting factor. Also in binding calcium to bone matrix. Important in bone healing. |

Therapeutic dose*—Best to obtain vitamin K from chlorophyll-rich foods and/or a fat-soluble chlorophyll supplement.

** NOTE: Do not use vitamin K if you are on blood-thinning drugs, such as Coumadin or Warfin. Vitamin K will interfere with their effects.

Adult RDA**—65–70 mcg.

Nutrient	Food Sources	Benefit Relative to Arthritis
Calcium	Dark green vegetables, carrots, brown rice, beans, almonds, walnuts, cabbage, oats, figs, dairy food.	The main mineral in bone tissue (especially the vertebrae of the spine, etc.).

Therapeutic dose*—500–1500 mg/day for arthritis

Adult RDA**—800–1200 mg.

Nutrient	Food Sources	Benefit Relative to Arthritis
Boron	Watermelon, tomatoes, apples, unfermented green teas.	Cell growth and essential in calcium metabolism.[19] Speeds healing of muscle tissue.

Therapeutic dose for arthritis—3–6 mg/day

No RDA.

Boron is beneficial in osteoarthritis. Five out of ten osteoarthritis patients showed significant improvement compared to placebo group when given 6 mg per day of boron.

Nutrient	Food Sources	Benefit Relative to Arthritis
Chromium	Brewer's yeast, whole wheat, nuts, liver, beets, mushrooms, fish, egg yolks.	Insulin regulation, glucose tolerance. Immune and circulatory system.

No specific therapeutic dose for arthritis.

Adult RDA**—.05–.2 mg

Nutrient	Food Sources	Benefit Relative to Arthritis
Cobalt	Organ meats, oysters, clams, milk.	Production of B_{12} and blood. Along with manganese, helps prevent viral infection.

No specific therapeutic dose for arthritis.

No RDA.

Nutrient	Food Sources	Benefit Relative to Arthritis
Copper	Seafood, eggs, almonds, legumes, whole wheat, pomegranates.	Synergist to vitamin C, enzyme activity, nervous system, liver support for detoxification, anti-inflammatory conditions

No specific therapeutic dose for arthritis.

Adult RDA**—2–3 mg; 1.5 to 3 mg/day for everyone over 11 years of age.

Iodine	Seafood, dulse, kelp, coastal vegetables.	Thyroid gland, hormone formation, metabolism, skin, hair, nails.

No specific therapeutic dose for arthritis.

Adult RDA**—150 mcg

Iron	Legumes, liver, oysters, dried fruit, whole grains, dark green vegetables.	Hemoglobin production, blood quality, muscle respiration, stress and disease resistance.

No specific therapeutic dose* for arthritis.

Adult RDA**—10–15 mg

Note: According to research, excessive iron in the diet can be detrimental. Men, especially, should be cautious about ingesting iron, because it can tend to increase oxidative damage and increased degenerative disease. Excess iron can accumulate in body tissue, including the joints, contributing to joint pain.

Nutrient	Food Sources	Benefit Relative to Arthritis
Magnesium	Raw, green vegetables (chlorophyll), raw wheat germ, sea food, apples.	Mineral metabolism, vitamin activity, calcium utilization, necessary catalyst for metabolic functions.
Therapeutic dose*—500 mg/day for arthritis. Adult RDA**—280–400 mg		
Manganese	Whole grains, egg yolk, nuts, seeds, green vegetables.	Bone hardening, connective tissue support (tendons and ligaments), enzyme activation.
Therapeutic dose*—34 mg/day for arthritis. Adult RDA**—2–5 mg/day		
Phosphorous	Whole grains, fish, meat, poul try, eggs, legumes, nuts, seeds, dairy products.	Bones, nervous system, energy production, cell growth and repair, calcium metabolism.
Therapeutic dose*—120 mg as ortho-phosphoric acid. Adult RDA**—1200 mg.		
Potassium	Greens, vegetables and fruit, whole grains, pota toes.	Proper water balance, growth, prevention of intestinal gas and constipation, aids in cases of gout and osteoarthritis by helping to keep proper acid-alkaline balance in blood and tissues.

Nutrient	Food Sources	Benefit Relative to Arthritis
Therapeutic dose*—500 mg/day for arthritis. Adult RDA**—1875–5625 mg		
Selenium	Seafood, whole grains, brewer's yeast.	Growth and repair. Teams with vitamin E, immune system.
No therapeutic dose for arthritis. Adult RDA**—50–70 mcg.		
Some Danish studies show selenium is low in individuals with rheumatoid arthritis.		
Silicon	Oats, apples and other fruits, rice, sunflower seeds, alfalfa, kelp, beets, onions; herbs such as horsetail grass; and oat, wheat or rice straw.	Bone growth and formation; connective tissue and ligament integrity, healing gastric ulcers.
Therapeutic dose*—20–30 mg/day for arthritis. No RDA**		
Sodium	Most all foods, sea salt, seafood.	Blood pH, stomach, nerves, muscles, water balance.
No therapeutic dose for arthritis. Adult RDA**—1100–3300 mg NOTE: excess sodium intake may contribute to excess urinary calcium loss.		

Nutrient	Food Sources	Benefit Relative to Arthritis
Sulphur	Cruciferous vegetables (cabbage, broccoli, cauliflower), carrots, eggs, radishes, garlic, onions, mustard, molasses, figs.	Needed as part of "protein infrastructure" of joint. Joint support and structure, adrenals, liver detoxification, component of B vitamins.

Therapeutic dose* for arthritis—consult health professional.

No RDA

Figs have sulphur compounds called ficins which reduce joint inflammation and swelling of soft tissue in rheumatoid arthritis.

Nutrient	Food Sources	Benefit Relative to Arthritis
Zinc[20]	Whole grains, wheat germ, seeds, brewer's yeast, nuts, spinach, mushrooms.	Wound healing, digestive enzymes, metabolism, skin. Effective in rheumatoid arthritis and diseases needing immune support.

Therapeutic dose*—consult health professional.

Adult RDA**—12-15 MG.

---

* Consult a health professional for proper recommendations on therapeutic doses. Best results are achieved when the proper balance of nutrients is used according to individual needs. Side effects are possible with high does of any single nutrient.

** U.S. government recommended dietary allowances (daily).

Powerful Proteolytic Enzymes

Potent enzymes—act as powerful anti-inflammatory and pain-controlling agents.
    —speed up "house cleaning" in injured and inflamed tissue.

The Dynamics of Inflammation:

When we are injured or when we are exposed to foreign toxic matter (i.e., viral infection), the body produces the chemical reactions called inflammation. Inflammation has, among other functions, the roles of:

1) housecleaning—cleaning out injury waste matter

2) protection—the area injured is closed off to keep foreign or toxic substances from invading other tissue.

Inflammation creates the symptoms of redness, heat, pain, swelling and, eventually, can interfere with range of motion. When the inflammatory process is occurring (i.e., housecleaning

> Proteolytic enzyme supplements are powerful tools to reduce inflammation, pain and swelling, allowing increased range of motion to improve joint health.

and protection), the repair mechanisms are slowed down or halted. So although inflammation serves some beneficial purpose, it needs to be controlled in order to:

1) allow repair of tissues

2) reduce or eliminate the pain and swelling

3) allow for an increased range of motion so that the arthritis process will not progress

**Enzymes control inflammation and pain
and support Repair!**

An effective enzyme supplement for fighting inflammation and pain contains the following ingredients:

pancreatin—100 mg. per tablet
bromelain—50 mg. per tablet
papain—50 mg. per tablet
amylase—10 mg. per tablet
lipase—10 mg. per tablet
trypsin and alpha chrmotrypsin—100 mg. per tablet

Preferably, these enzymes will be combined in one product. The dosage will depend on the individual product and its quality and potencies. Generally, for acute inflammation—10 tabs, 5 times per day *without food* on *an empty stomach*; then as inflammation and pain are reduced, 5 tabs, 4 times per day *without food, on an empty stomach.*

Our bodies naturally produce proteolytic (protein digesting) enzymes to digest foods, for metabolism and to help regulate many components of *inflammation.*

Enzymes accelerate the housecleaning of injury waste matter. Using supplements of proteolytic enzymes *between meals on an empty stomach* is like sending in extra power vacuums and to assist the reduction of inflammation time and allow the rejuvenation (healing and repair) process to accelerate.

Chlorophyll

Chlorophyll, the green pigment in plants, is abundant in such plants as kale, spinach, parsley, broccoli, the green leafy parts of barley and wheat grass, etc., and has many blood-cleansing and building properties. Chlorophyll also destroys guanidine, an irritant produced by damaged tissue, such as that produced by arthritis. Guanidine is a very alkaline substance found with bowel toxicity and constipation.

Chlorophyll is rich in fat-soluble vitamins, magnesium (a catalyst in many enzyme reactions) and is helpful in maintaining the body's acid-alkaline balance. Chlorophyll's unique properties also help to release stored iron from the liver and assists in the conversion of iron into the hemoglobin molecule. Chlorophyll has anti-bacteria and anti-viral properties. One of nature's best natural anti- inflammatory agents, chlorophyll helps reduce the pain and inflammation of arthritis.

Green juice from your barley has a strong anti-inflammatory effect, according to research reported at the 101st annual meeting of the Japan Pharmacological Society in 1981.

Try to eat raw, dark-green vegetables daily. You may also juice raw vegetables for concentrations of the nutrients from wheat grass, parsley and barley greens. Cooking dark green plants destroys chlorophyll, so emphasize raw or lightly cooked greens.

If you use a chlorophyll supplement, always select the fat-soluble and not the water-soluble (or processed) capsules. Fat-soluble chlorophyll supplements have the anti-oxidants (vitamins E and K, vitamin A as carotenoids, magnesium and iron all present in the plant to guard it against destruction). The water-soluble capsules do not have these anti-oxidants.

Alfalfa

Alfalfa, a plant usually classified as an herb, is rich in vitamins A, B, E, D and K as well as minerals and protein. Alfalfa has eight essential amino acids needed for food assimilation. In fact, the Arabic translation of this beneficial herb's name means "the father of all foods."

Alfalfa is known to help relieve osteoarthritis stiffness and pain, stomach distress and edema. Some natural food supplements contain alfalfa, and you can also use whole alfalfa tablets, and alfalfa teas in moderation, and alfalfa sprouts.

In rheumatoid arthritis and other immune system disorders, *alfalfa supplements are NOT recommended* due to evidence revealing how alfalfa supplements can interfere and suppress immune function in individuals with an already compromised immune system.[21] Please remember that not all foods or supplements are beneficial to everyone. It is always important to consider individual needs.

Brewer's Yeast

Brewer's yeast, a nonleavening yeast, is one of the best sources of B vitamins and is also high in minerals, enzymes, amino acids and RNA (ribonucleic acid, which is beneficial to the immune system).

High in phosphorous, brewer's yeast can be used in arthritic conditions where phosphorous is too low, causing calcium to precipitate out of the blood and into the joints.

Brewer's yeast can be added to foods as powder or flakes and it also is available in tablet form or as part of whole-food supplements.

Kelp

Kelp, one of the many forms of seaweed, is a rich source of minerals, especially calcium, iodine and magnesium. It is also high in the vitamin B complex, as well as vitamins D, E and K. Kelp is beneficial for arthritis and is used in a tablet or powdered form or as a seasoning for food.

Adrenal Support

When you're seeking help for arthritis, it is important to consider possible need of adrenal support. These two small glands, only weighing about 3 to 5 grams, are located above the kidneys. They have one of the highest rates of blood flow in the body and contain the highest level of vitamin C per gram in the body.

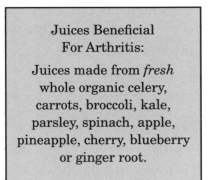

Juices Beneficial For Arthritis:

Juices made from *fresh* whole organic celery, carrots, broccoli, kale, parsley, spinach, apple, pineapple, cherry, blueberry or ginger root.

The adrenal glands provide an anti-stress and anti-inflammatory effect for the body, producing adrenaline and other hormones, like corticosteroids. The adrenal glands are usually overworked with joint pain, chronic inflammation, heavy-metal toxicity, allergies and emotional stress.

Symptoms of low adrenal function may include dizziness, fatigue, low blood pressure, allergies, respiratory weakness, low blood sugar problems and muscle and joint pain.

Early Signs of Possible Low Adrenal Function:

1. chronic weakness and fatigue
2. allergy sensitivity reactions
3. asthmatic type symptoms
4. low blood pressure
5. reactive low blood sugar
6. inflammation
7. muscle and joint pain
8. poor memory
9. sleep disturbances
10. any chronic illness (infections, virus, etc.)

In addition to symptom patterns and appropriate blood tests for adrenal function evaluations, your health professional can check for low adrenal function (hypoadrenia) by doing a Ragland Postural Blood Pressure Test (see following). Also, appropriate laboratory work includes: serum potassium and sodium (potassium may be elevated with a low sodium); renin, cortisol, aldosterone (renin may be increased and cortisol and aldosterone decreased); and/or a DHEA saliva or blood test (please see Appendix I for laboratories offering adrenal stress tests).

The adrenal glands synthesize over 150 different hormones; one of the most publicized is DHEA (dehydroepiandrosterone), one of the steroid hormones. Some studies suggest that DHEA supplementation could be effective treatment for immune system disorders, such as rheumatoid arthritis and lupus. However, most testing has been done on laboratory animals and human studies have not been able to show conclusively that DHEA has long-term benefits.

As with any hormonal support, caution should always be taken. Verification of need should be determined by a physician's analysis of DHEA levels through a blood or saliva test before taking a DHEA supplement. There have been reported side effects of taking DHEA when not needed or if taken in excess. As the saying goes, "don't try to fix something that isn't broken." Remember, health programs are based on *individual* needs and *not* on "the supplement of the month club"—"fix-all," "quick-fix" hype.

RAGLUND POSTURAL BLOOD PRESSURE TEST

Recumbent Blood Pressure:

1. Lie down for at least three minutes and have your systolic (the top number) blood pressure taken.

Standing Blood Pressure:

2. Pump the blood pressure cuff up again and prior to standing up. Once the cuff has been pumped up again, stand up and have the systolic measurement read again.

Interpretation:

3. With the normal adrenal function, there should be an increase of 6 mm to 10 mm of the systolic blood pressure from the recumbent to the standing reading. With the low adrenal function, the standing reading will be equal to or less than the recumbent.

In addition, the overall systolic blood pressure should be 100 mm–130 mm.

Nutritional support for low adrenal function may include:

1. Vitamins A and C complexes.

2. Pantothenic acid, thiamine pyrophosphate and the other members of the entire B complex. Pantothenic acid is part of the B complex and is found in brewer's yeast, egg yolks, whole grains and organ meats. Thiamine pyrophosphate, vitamin B_1, is found in whole grains, brewer's yeast, nuts, liver, beef and pork. Green beans, celery, zucchini, onions and tomatoes are also helpful for adrenal support.

3. Essential fatty acids and the co-factors B_6, zinc and magnesium.

4. Protomorphogen supplements (natural tissue glandular extracts) containing DNA, RNA and other adrenal material or fractions to support adrenals.[22]

5. Avoiding caffeine, excess alcohol, cigarette smoking and refined carbohydrates also helps to support adrenal function.

Thyroid Support

The thyroid gland, another team member of the endocrine system, regulates our metabolic rate and influences calcium utilization and fat mobilization. The thyroid is a tiny butterfly-shaped gland in your neck which wraps around the windpipe. The thyroid releases the hormone thyroxine that regulates about every organ in your body. In fact, the entire endocrine system is involved with calcium utilization and proper acid-alkaline balance of the body either directly or indirectly, so it is important to have good hormonal balance and not to single out or isolate one gland as more important than another.

With arthritis, the thyroid and adrenal glands are usually considered first for possible need of nutritional support. Experts feel thyroid problems go undetected for years and estimate two percent of women have hyper (overactive) thyroid and ten percent of all women have hypo (underactive) thyroids. Hormones made in the thyroid are essential to normal metabolism and the growth and maintenance of major organs and muscles.

Signs of hypo (low) thyroidism can include:	Signs of hyper (overactive) thyroidism can include:
fatigue — mood swings sensitivity to cold — weight gain dry skin — hair loss	weight loss — heat sensitivity heart palpitations — vision problems — irritability

In conjunction with your symptom history, your physician will confirm your thyroid function by analyzing a thyroid profile blood test including: TSH, T_3, T_4. The TSH blood test is actually a measure of anterior pituitary function. Since your anterior pituitary and your thyroid work in a feedback partnership, an elevated TSH can indicate low thyroid function, whereas a low TSH can indicate a need for anterior pituitary support.

A preliminary test to rule out either an underactive or an overactive endocrine function is the Broda Barnes Test developed by Broda Barnes, M.D.[23] Dr. Barnes and many other physicians found that thyroid blood tests did not always reveal subclinical or borderline underactive thyroid problems which would then signal a need for further investigation of which gland (thyroid or adrenal, for example) needs support within the endocrine system. They found that a resting underarm temperature below 97.8°F can indicate low endocrine function. An underarm temperature above 98.2°F can indicate high endocrine dysfunction.

Nutritional support[24] for an imbalance in the thyroid can include:

1. L-Tyrosine (an amino acid).

2. Protomorphogen supplements (natural tissue glandular extracts) containing DNA, RNA and other thyroid materials or fractions.[25]

3. Copper, zinc, B_6, B_{12}, folic acid and betaine.

4. Organic iodine.

5. Celtic sea salt—contains a natural balance of trace-mineral components healthful for your thyroid. (Order from: Grain and Salt Society, 1-800-867-7258 or check with your local health food co-op or store).

Consult a qualified health professional for exact doses, because individual needs vary. Prescribed thyroid medication and many other medications should be adjusted by your physician to avoid any risks of withdrawal symptoms. **Never** discontinue any prescribed medications without your physician's advice. Certain individuals with low or high thyroid conditions require a prescribed thyroid medication, so work with your physician on your individual needs.

Hormone balance (endocrine balance) is vital to the function of your body chemistry and so its intricate complexities should be treated with respect and care.

Homeopathy

Homeopathy, a system of health care originating in the 18th century, is practiced worldwide, especially in Europe. Today, homeopathy is gaining credence in the United States as a valuable tool in health care since it is based on treatment of the whole body.

A homeopathic remedy consists of plant nutrients (botanicals and herbs) as biological materials combined in a titrated formula (simply put—"minute doses"). Modern-day homeopathics, produced under laboratory conditions, are safe, effective and have no side effects when used correctly. Remedies may be in pill, liquid, injection form or found in ointments or creams.

Under the principles of homeopathy, specific detoxification remedies are first used to assist in the detoxification, or cleansing, of organs and systems (lymphatics, liver, kidney, intestines, etc.). A homeopathic remedy may next be used for the "rebuilding" of cells and tissues. The most commonly used homeopathics for arthritis are:

1. *Arnica* (leopard's bane) useful for relief of pain. Is generally used for the initial relief of pain and bruising caused from surgery or injury. It can be taken before or after surgery to reduce pain and bruising. Available in oral or ointment forms.

2. *Bryonia* (wild hops)—for joint swelling, inflammation and redness.

3. *Rhustox* (poison ivy)—for pain and stiffness around the joints and ligaments when symptoms are worse in cold weather or are worse with inactivity.

Follow the directions from the manufacturer or more importantly, your health care professional. Most homeopathic remedies are taken 15 minutes before or 30 minutes after eating, brushing your teeth or drinking anything other than pure water.

Homeopathy is a complex system and requires the experience of a health professional versed in using homeopathic remedies which are complementary with other health care systems for arthritis. Please refer to appendices I and III for resource information.

Natural Anti-inflammatory Agents, Anti-oxidant Support and Pain Controllers

Rheumatoid arthritis is considered an auto-immune disease where the immune response is directed against the body's own tissue, thus causing inflammatory reactions which eventually damage body structures. In osteoarthritis, inflammation is not usually present, but there is joint destruction, stiffness and pain. Whole food supplements containing nutrients with their synergists work to support the body chemistry in the most ideal way and complement healthy food choices. Remember that *no single nutrient works alone* to help correct nutritional imbalance.

How free radical damage contributes to arthritis:

1. Normal body chemistry processes, injury, toxic environmental chemical exposure (smoking & food additives, etc.) and inflammation all produce free radical damage.
2. The body uses protective enzymes, hundreds of different anti-oxidants from foods and metabolites to fight oxidation and free radical damage.
3. In arthritis, the body cannot adequately fight free radical damage without these nutrients and so cells, tissues and organs become damaged.

A Reference List of Natural Anti-inflammatory Agents, Anti-oxidant Support and Pain Controllers

Boswellia **(Ayurvedic herb)** or **Boswellian (extract of Boswellia)**—follow dosages recommended on package. Useful for pain and inflammation control.

Bromelain **(enzyme from pineapple)**—as a supplement, used for its **anti-inflammatory and pain-control benefits**. Take 5 to 6 capsules, 5 times daily on empty stomach. See, also, information under **Proteolytic Enzymes** in this chapter.

Anti-inflammatory foods:

Small pickles (gherkins),[*] raspberries,[*] paprika,[*] prunes,[*] blueberries,[*] cherries,[*] curry powder,[*] dried dates,[*]

Cantaloupe, whole grains, pineapple, sage, figs, celery, cruciferous vegetables (broccoli, cauliflower, etc.) apples, black currants, sweet potatoes, garlic, carrots.

Marine fish (cod, salmon, etc.) and flaxseeds sources of omega 3 fatty acids; ginger root.

[*]These foods have anti-inflammatory effects due to their natural salicylates (aspirin's anti-inflammatory effect is due to salicylate content)

Capsaicin (capsicum minimum)—a natural extract of hot chili peppers (cayenne)—Capsaicin blocks the brain chemical (substance P) involved in the transmission of pain signals and increases the body's production of pain killers called endorphins. Capsaicin extract-containing ointments or lotions can be rubbed into areas of pain around the joint. Also, soaking a gauze cloth in hot pepper sauce containing cayenne and then **applying to painful area may relieve pain**.

Pain control and reduction of inflammation

Enzyme therapy is beneficial in reducing inflammation, swelling and tissue trauma. Enzyme therapy aids in removing waste products from the inflammed joints. Complementary to enzyme therapy is immune support.

Cat's Claw (**Uña de gato**)—1 to 6 grams daily or 1 to 2 cups of tea form. Helpful for **pain relief**. Do *not* use with pregnancy or lactation.

Celery seed—2 capsules of celery seed extract or celery (4 stalks daily)—contains numerous **anti-inflammatory** compounds (phytochemicals).

Curcumin[26] (**Cucuma longa**)—found in turmeric, the spice made into curry and yellow mustard; 400 to 600 mg, 3 times per day or follow package directions. Or 2 1/2 teaspoons, 3 times daily in juice. Useful in **pain control**.

Feverfew (**Tanacetum parthenium**)—1 to 2 capsules, 2 times daily. The theory of feverfew's benefit is that it may block hormones that are involved in pain process. Useful for **pain control**.

Ginger root—5 grams daily or one of the following: 1 capsule, 2 times daily; 1/3 teaspoon ground ginger, 3 times daily; or 1 teaspoon freshly ground ginger root 3 times daily. Can be used in cooking or used in a tea or herbal capsule form. Can **reduce joint stiffness or swelling. Can be as effective as NSAIDs (non-steroidal anti-inflammatory drugs).**

GLA (**gamma linolenic acid**)—2,800 mg per day (found in product supplements of capsules containing plant sources of black current seed oil and primrose oil) long-term supplementation effective in **reducing rheumatoid arthritis pain**.[27] Act as **anti-inflammatory** and **immune support**.

Green Teas—found in health food stores, co-ops, and oriental markets. A tea drink used by ancient China since 3000 B.C.; **anti-oxidant activity** and supplies vitamins A, K and B complex.

Niacinamide (B₃)—500 mg, 2 times daily. Increase as needed in 500 mg. increments up to 2000 mg. maximum per day to **relieve stiffness and pain**.

Oligomeric Proanthrocyanidins (OPCs)—50 mg, 3 to 4 times daily. A highly specialized group of bioflavinoids with anti-oxidant effects up to 50 times more potent than Vit. E and up to 20 times more powerful than Vit. C. **Pycnogenol**® is registered trademark name of the maritime pine bark extract of OPCs.[28] **Grapeseeds** or **Pips** are also abundant sources of OPC compounds.

Omega 3 fatty acids **(flaxseed and deep-ocean fish oils)**— 2 to 4 tbsp. daily or 3 to 6 capsules daily for **anti-inflammatory and immune support**.

Quercitin **(a flavinoid compound found in onions and garlic)**—a **potent anti-oxidant**. Can be found in whole food supplements, also.

Inflammation, characteristic of rheumatoid arthritis and joint destruction found in osteoarthritis can be reduced in many cases by the use of **Super Oxide Dismutase**, pycnogenol and other anti-oxidants (including vitamins A, C and E and their synergists). These agents help reduce free-radical pathology associated with inflammation in the synovial fluid of the joints. **Super Oxide Dismutase**, pycnogenol and other anti-oxidants are used by health care professionals to reduce inflammation in rheumatoid arthritis and also reduce the cartilage and bone wear, tear and damage of osteoarthritis. The beneficial dose of **Super Oxide Dismutase** is 50 mcg to 1000 mcg daily, depending on need.

Analgesics—**Natural Pain Killers (analgesics)**—can help block body's perception of pain.

chili peppers	ginger	onion	garlic
clove	licorice	peppermint	

L-histidine (an amino acid) is often low in individuals with arthritis.* Food sources include:

Organic eggs dried peas and beans whole grains
wheat germ   brown rice   nutritional yeast
soybeans

According to Donald A. Gerben, associate professor of medicine at Down-state Medical Center in New York.

Anti-oxidants

Glutathione—anti-aging anti-oxidant! Enhances immune system and squelches free radicals

- asparagus—1/2 cup—26.3 mg.
- avocado—1/2—31.3 mg.
- grapefruit—1/2—14.6 mg.
- potato—7 oz.—12.7 mg.
- pumpkin or winter squash—1/2 cup—14.4 mg.
- tomato—4 oz.—10.9 mg.
- water melon—1 cup—28.3 mg.

Recommended amount is 25 to 50 mg per day. A University of Michigan Study revealed that people over 60 with high levels of gluthathione had less arthritis, heart disease and diabetes.

Anti-oxidants Protect and Reverse Osteoarthritis
A study done by the Framingham osteoarthritis Cohort Study revealed that high intake of anti-oxidant nutrients may reduce the *risk* of cartilage loss and progression of pain and the disease in osteoarthritis.

McAlindon, T.E., et al.: Do anti-oxidant micro nutrients protect against the development and progression of knee arthritis? Arthritis & Rheumatism, 39: 648–56, 1996.

Anti-oxidants—These nutrients protect against free radical (unstable oxygen molecules) damage. Research shows that individuals with low levels of anti-oxidants such as vitamins E and C, selenium, beta carotene) had increased rates of rheumatoid arthritis[29] and other degenerative diseases. There are hundreds of anti-oxidants in foods, many still being isolated and studied for their benefits.

Summary: Anti-oxidants are fighters of free radical production. Our bodies have a natural anti-free radical system that can fight degenerative diseases like osteoarthritis and rheumatoid arthritis, but we must supply the nutrients to keep these systems in check. Research will continue to investigate the numerous functions and supplemental therapies to rejuvenate the body.

NOTES

15. Setuikar 1, Giachen C, Zanolo G. Absorption distribution and excretion of radioactivity after a single intravenous or oral administration of (14C) glucosamine to the rat. Pharmatherapeutica 1984; 3:538–555.

16. Morrison, M. Therapeutic applications of chondroitin-4-sulfate. Appraisal of biological properties. Folia Angiologica 1977; 25:225–233.

17. McAlindon, et. al. *Arthritis and Rheumatism*, 4/96; 39(4): 648–656.

18. Sperling, Dr. Richard, *Arthritis and Rheumatism*, 9/87. (30:988–997).

19. Travers, Richard L., M.D., et al. *Clinical Pearls*, 1991. Edit. (pg. 86).

20. The effects of sulphur and zinc are examined by Carl C. Pfeiffer, Ph.D., M.D., in the book *Zinc and Other Micro-Nutrients*, New York.

21. Herbert V. Kasdan TS, "Alfalfa, Vitamin E and Autoimmune Disorders." *American Journal of Clinical Nutrition.* 1994; 60:639–40.

22. Schmid, F. and Stein, J. (ed). *Cell Research and Cellular Therapy.* Thoune, Switzerland: Ott Publishers, 1967.

23. Barnes, Broda, M.D., *Hypothyroidism*, New York: Thomas Y. Crowell Pub., 1976.

24. Boers, et al., and Wright, Jonathon V., M.D., *New England Journal of Medicine,* Vol. 313, Sept. 1985. (pp 709–715).

25. Schmid, F. and Stein, J. (ed.). Cell Research and Cellular Therapy. Thoune, Switzerland: Ott Publishers, 1967.

26. Goud, V. K. et. al. "Effect of Tumeric on Xenobiotic Metabolizing Enzymes." *Plant Foods Hum Nutr* 1993; 44(1) 87–92.

27. Zurier, et al., *Arthritis and Rheumatism*, 11/96; 39 (11): 1808–1817.

28. Masquelier, J. United States Patent No. 4, 698, 366. Oct. 6, 1987.

29. Darlington, L.G., *Dietary Therapy for Arthritis Nutrition and Rheumatic Diseases*, 1991: 17(2): 273–85.

"There is no healing force outside the body."

—Isaac Jennings

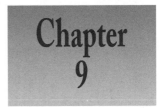
A Master Plan for Osteoarthritis and Knee and Back Injuries

Osteo-arthritis, degenerative joint disease, is primarily diagnosed by noting symptoms of joint pain and stiffness, especially in the morning and in cold weather.

The joints may be swollen and deformed with bone overgrowth (spurs). Proper diagnoses are made with X-rays and a complete history of symptoms.

Refer to Chapters 3, 4 and 5—especially information under liver and bowel support

The following "Master Plan" Nutrition Program for osteoarthritis is also beneficial for individuals seeking breakthrough healing for knee and back injury and pain (cartilage, ligament and tendon support).

Glucosamine Sulfates: 500 mg—3 times daily × 8 weeks; then 500 mg daily for maintenance. (See Chapter 8.)

Purified chondroitin sulfates: 600 mg—3 times daily. Chondroitin sulfates are potent, anti-inflammatory, anti-stiffness support; enhance repair of cartilage and inhibit degradation of cartilage.

A whole organic food supplement as a source of vitamins, minerals, enzymes, anti-oxidants and other factors that support bone, cartilage growth and repair. (See Chapter 8)

Proteolytic Enzyme Product: (The following ingredients are combined in one supplement)

Bromelain, 50–100 mg per tablet
Pancreatin, 100 mg per tablet
Papain, 10–50 mg per tablet
Chymotrypsin and Trypsin, 100 mg per tablet
Amylase, 10 mg per tablet
Lipase, 10 mg. per tablet

—4 tablets, 3 times daily and 4 at bedtime—*taken on an empty stomach between meals*. (See Chapter 8 for information on Proteolytic Enzymes)

Calcium glycerophosphate: 850 mg per tablet **and orthophosphoric acid:** 395 mg per tablet; 3 tablets, 3 times per day. Combined in one supplement with inositol, 20 mg per tablet (to support calcium to phosphorous balance; aides in dissolving bone spurs).

Your physician can monitor the blood calcium to phosphorous ratio by comparing your blood calcium number to the phosphorous. When the ratio is not the ideal 10 parts calcium to 4 parts phosphorous, it can indicate a need for either calcium or phosphorous or an assimilation problem.

Flaxseed oil capsules: 3 to 6 capsules per day or 6 tablespoons daily.
(Refer to Chapter 3 [fats] and Chapter 8.)

Calcium citrate: 60 mg—3 times daily (if needed, for improving calcium and magnesium balance.)
Your physician can analyze your need for calcium through a blood test of your calcium and phosphorous ratio. The blood calcium to blood phosphorous should be 10 parts calcium to 4 parts phosphorous. If the ratio is "weighted" to the phosphorous, calcium is needed.

Horsetail (herbs): 1 tablet, 3 times daily (440 mg per day)
A source of silicon; helps with calcium absorption.

Breakthroughs in Natural Healing involves the principles of total nutrition outlined in Chapters 3 through 8. Please review this valuable support information. In summary, strive to achieve these goals:

1. Drink at least 8 to 10 glasses of pure water daily.

2. Increase raw, fresh organic fruits and vegetables in diet.

3. Eliminate or reduce hydrogenated or partially hydrogenated fats. Use raw (cold pressed) oils and fats (e.g., flaxseed, sesame seed, olive oil, etc.).

4. Reduce or eliminate processed/refined carbohydrates, alcohol and caffeine (coffee, tea, chocolate and sodas).

5. *Avoid* calcium carbonate supplements and *anti-acids* (calcium carbonate is poorly absorbed and anti-acids can contain aluminum and interfere with good digestion).

Osteoarthritis

This chapter contains a "Master Plan" for nutritional support of osteoarthritis and even healing support for back and knee pain and injuries. To discover the entire breakthroughs in natural healing, please read Chapters 12 through 16. You will learn some valuable information in healing using exercise manipulative therapy, acupuncture, healing touch and mind-body techniques. Integration of as many methods as possible allows for breakthrough rejuvenation and healing for arthritis relief.

"The key to a strong, healthy immune system is optimal nutrition."

—Leo Galland, M.D.

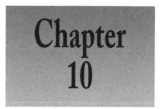

Chapter 10

A Master Plan for Rheumatoid Arthritis

Rheumatoid arthritis (RA) is diagnosed by your physician by obtaining a complete history of your symptoms and blood test analysis.

Doctors diagnose RA by analyzing blood tests, including an Erythrocyte Sedimentation Rate (ESR) and/or a positive Rheumatoid Factor (RF) and X-rays. In some cases where individuals have a negative rheumatoid factor in their blood test, rheumatoid arthritis may still be present. So it is important to give your physician your complete medical symptom history, so she or he can properly diagnose your condition.

> Rheumatoid arthritis is considered an autoimmune disease. The immune system may not really be low or weak . . . but may actually be disorganized.

Symptoms of rheumatoid arthritis include:

a) morning stiffness

b) inflammation in three or more joint areas

c) rheumatoid nodules

Traditionally, RA is treated with aspirin (salicylates), non-steroidal anti-inflammatory drugs, gold compounds, penicillamine corticosteroids and, with severe joint damage, surgery.

The following strategies for supporting your body chemistry holistically are not necessarily meant to replace a physician's treatment program for RA, but can be used complementarily. Consult with your health professional to design a comprehensive treatment program.

In RA, the immune system is not really low or weak; it may actually be disorganized. Investigate (meaning: rule out) these conditions which may play a role in upsetting or unbalancing your nutritional state (including digestion, assimilation, metabolism) and affecting your overall immune system and body chemistry. A rheumatoid arthritis may be aggravated by:

1. A viral condition. Your health professional can order a complete blood count (white blood cell, neutrophil, lymphocytes, eosinophil) to ascertain if there is a "viral pattern." If the lymphocyte count is elevated and the white blood count and neutrophils are low or marginally low, this may indicate a viral condition.

2. A bacterial infection. Your health professional will order a Complete Blood Count and Differential blood chemistry.

3. Food sensitivities which contribute to inflammation in the body.

See Chapter 4 on programs to investigate and rule out food sensitivities. Digestive distress and intestinal permeability (dysbiosis) may cause undigested proteins, bacteria and possible yeast components to be absorbed or leak through the bowel wall, contributing to inflamma tory reactions.

Some people with RA benefit from removing all dairy products and grains containing gluten (all grains except rice, millet and corn). Consider avoiding these foods for a minimum of ten days and watch for symptomic change. (See Chapter 4.)

4. Parasites in the bowel or as a systemic (affecting the body) amoebic condition may also compromise the immune system.

   Tests: *Comprehensive Stool and Digestive Analysis* and a *White Blood Count Differential.* With parasites, the blood level of monocytes, basophils and eosinophils will be elevated in the white blood count differential. Please refer to laboratory information in Appendix I..

5. Yeast (candida).

   Evaluated by a positive *stool analysis* (*Comprehensive Stool and Digestive Analysis*) for yeast overgrowth or a positive *candida antigen test* found through a blood test (see Appendix I).

6. Digestive dysfunction due to low hydrochloric acid (hypochlorhydria) creating insufficient protein breakdown, gastro-intestinal irritants and eventually inflammation (see Chapter 3 for program to support digestive distress).

7. Heavy metal body burden—an abnormal tissue level of aluminum, cadmium, mercury, and lead may compromise the immune system's function and also compete with the role of beneficial minerals in the body (for example, aluminum toxicity competes with calcium absorption). A *hair analysis* can measure and rule out heavy metal body burdens of toxic metals.

8. Genetic pre-disposition.

Refer to appendix I for the laboratories suggested recommended to complete of a Comprehensive Stool and Digestive Analysis, hair analysis and blood chemistries. Your health professional will order these laboratory tests and work with you to determine your special needs. If your health professional finds a need to support any of the above conditions, they can outline individualized and specialized holistic treatment using enzyme therapy, homeopathic and specific nutritional supplements.

Magnesium, calcium, selenium, boron, potassium, manganese, and iodine are often needed as nutrients to support RA. Most of these nutrients act as cofactors that stimulate enzymatic reactions to regulate the metabolism of linoleic acid and linolenic acid. The essential fatty acids are vital in promoting the formation of a beneficial level of prostaglandins involved with controlling the inflammation and immune system reactions. These nutrients also regulate the activity of white blood cells, T cells and B cells.

In the Midwestern states, copper is often low in soils and therefore in plant foods. So, copper supplementation may also be helpful in RA. Copper needs can be determined by the blood tests: *Serum Copper* and *Ceruloplasm (Copper Binding Protein)*.

A "Master Plan" Nutritional Program for Rheumatoid Arthritis:

1. **A whole organic food supplement designed as *broad* spectrum immune system and tissue support** containing enzymes; antioxidants; minerals manganese, copper, magnesium; trace minerals selenium, boron (taken with meals). (See also, Chapter 8.)

2. **Thymus Protomorphogen Supplement** (natural tissue glandular extracts) containing DNA, RNA and other thymic material or fractions.[29]

The thymus gland, located at the base of the neck, produces a hormone called thymosin that enhances the immune system. According to a university study and clinical studies, it is proven that thymus gland extract products taken orally actually do stimulate thymosin production.[30]

In 1992, Carson B. Burgstiner, M.D., board certified obstetrician-gynecologist and past president of the Medical Association of Georgia, reported in the *Journal of the Medical Association of Georgia* his personal experience with using thymus extracts to "cure his hepatitis." He later headed a university study to verify the benefits of thymus tissue extracts. He believes thymus therapy can benefit people with almost any immune challenge, including lupus and rheumatoid arthritis.

3. **Super Oxide Dismutase (SOD)**—30 mg, 3 times daily (or 10,000 units 3 times daily) taken with meals. SOD is an enzyme that breaks down the superoxide free radical, acting as a potent anti-oxidant. (See also, Chapter 8.)

4. **Proteolytic enzyme product** (the following ingredients are combined in one supplement) for anti-inflammatory and pain-control support.

   Bromelain—50 to 100 mg per tab
   Papain—10 to 50 mg per tab
   Amylase—10 mg per tab
   Lipase—10 mg per tab
   Pancreatin 400 mg per tab
   Chymotrypsin and trypsin—100 mg per tab

   4 tabs—3 times per daily and 4 at bedtime—*taken on an empty stomach between meals* (See Chapter 8.)

5. **Flaxseed oil and/or black current seed oil**—3 to 6 capsules per day or 6 tablespoons per day—with meals.

6. **Chondroitin sulfates**—300 mg—3 times daily with food (ideally, purified chondroitin sulfates) and **glucosamine sulfates**

   Chondroitin sulfates help modulate ("balance") the immune system so the body's immune system will reorganize itself and not attack its own tissue. Chondroitin sulfates offer potent anti-inflammatory, anti-stiffness and pain-controlling support; and heal the joint cartilage. (See Chapters 7 and 8.)

7. Liver support, if needed (see Chapter 5 for liver support)

8. Adrenal support, if needed (see Chapter 8 for adrenal support)

9. Homeopathic support (see Chapter 6 for homeopathic support)

Team Members to the "Master Plan"

As needed on an individualized basis:

1. Digestive support product containing:
   hydrochloric acid
   glutamic acid
   pepsin, ammonium chloride, B6
   (See Chapter 3)

2. Amino acid/protein supplement, to heal tissue and maintain healthy joint and muscle tissue.

3. B_{12} and folate (folic acid) support

   The best method to determine a B12 need is through a blood test called methyl melonic acid; consult with your physician for laboratory analysis of need.

4. L-histidine—3 times daily with food
   (a beneficial amino acid)
   Ideally as L-histidine—the naturally free form of histidine

Breakthrough Natural Healing involves the principles of total nutrition outlined in Chapters 3 through 8. Please review the valuable support information. In summary, strive to achieve these goals:

1. Drink at least 8 to 10 glasses of pure water daily.

2. Increase raw, fresh, organic fruits and vegetables in diet.

3. Eliminate hydrogenated or partially hydrogenated fats. Use raw (cold pressed) oils and fats (e.g., flaxseed, sesame seed, olive oil, etc.)

4. Reduce or eliminate processed/refined carbohydrates, alcohol and caffeine containing foods (coffee, tea, chocolate and sodas).

This chapter contains the "Master Plan" for nutritional support of rheumatoid arthritis. To discover the entire Breakthroughs in Natural Healing, please read on. You will learn some valuable tools in healing using exercise, manipulative therapy, acupuncture, healing touch and mind-body techniques. Integration of as many methods as possible allows for breakthrough rejuvenation and healing for arthritis relief.

NOTES

29. Burgstiner, Carson B., M.D., *Journal of the Medical Association of Georgia*, 1/91; 80(1): 21–22.

"The key to the ability to change is a changeless sense of who you are, what you are about and what you value."

—Stephen R. Covey

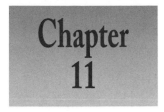

Special Nutritional Recommend- ations for Gouty Arthritis

Gout affects approximately one million Americans, and most of these afflictions occur in men.

Gout is an arthritic condition where high amounts of uric acid accumulate in the joints and blood. Elevated uric acid, a by-product of protein metabolism in the body, can stress the kidneys and liver, as well as the joints. The control of gout, therefore, is aimed at decreasing the uric acid levels in the body. Diet plays a major role in this treatment.

Special instructions:

1. Avoid high-fat foods (a high-fat diet retards the excretion of uric acid). Avoid fried foods. Limit fat to 20% to 25% of daily calories.

2. Drink two to three quarts of liquid daily to help dilute urinary uric acid (water is the liquid of choice). As discussed earlier, distilled water can be used during the treatment program. Uric acid is excreted from the body by the kidneys, so drinking sufficient quantities of water daily helps your kidneys efficiently excrete uric acid so that it will not accumulate in the blood or joints.

3. Avoid all alcohol, including beer and wine. Alcohol will aggravate gout mainly because it is metabolized like fat and retards excretion of uric acid.

4. Avoid foods with a high purine content (150-800 mg of purine nitrogen per 100 grams of food). High purine (especially high in pork and red meat) creates high uric-acid levels, since it is the precursor of uric acid in protein metabolism. Foods to avoid include:

   - pork
   - beef—all red meat
   - organ meats (liver, kidney, sweetbreads, etc.)
   - anchovies, herring, mackerel, scallops, lobster
   - wild game, goose
   - luncheon/processed meats
   - meat broths, drippings, extracts, gravies
   - mincemeat (containing meat or meat by-products)
   - brewer's and baker's yeast

5. Limit foods with moderate purine content (50-150 mg of purine nitrogen per 100 grams of food).

   No more than four ounces/day of one of the following:
   - fish—avoid those listed in #4 above
   - poultry—avoid those listed in #4 above
   - seafood—avoid those listed in #4 above (emphasize marine or cold-water fish such as salmon, cod, haddock, tuna, etc.)

6. Avoid tea, coffee, chocolate and cocoa—all of which also contain purine components.

7. Avoid refined sugar and flour.

8. Avoid citrus juice (orange and grapefruit).

9. Avoid excess sodium.

10. Select a diet high in:

   a. Fresh fruits and vegetables (except those listed in #4 above). Eat daily fruits and vegetables high in vitamins A and C. Red sour cherries, black cherries and strawberries (fresh, frozen or juiced) are beneficial for helping reduce uric acid levels. Potassium-rich foods (potatoes, bananas, dark greens and other fruits and vegetables) also help in prevention and treatment of gout.

   b. Whole grains—avoid processed or refined grains as much as possible.

   c. Lean animal protein—small servings as listed in #5 above

   d. High-quality fats (cold-pressed oils, such as flaxseed oil and olive oil; raw nuts and seeds). Limit amounts to less than 25% of total daily calories.

11. Men, especially, have an increased risk of developing gout if overweight. If you need to lose weight, do so slowly. Rapid weight loss may aggravate gouty arthritis.

12. Supplemental support—using whole organic concentrates (made from raw, biologically active ingredients).

Daily:

   (a) folic acid—1600 mcg, 4 times per day with food until pain and swelling is gone; then 800 mcg—3 times per day with food.

- B complex (see nutrient chart in Chapter 8)
- vitamin C complex (up to 5000 mg)
- multiple vitamin and mineral supplement
- alfalfa tablets (10-15 tablets)
- vitamin E complex (400–1200 I.U.)

   (b)
- potassium and trace minerals (alkaline-ash minerals). Potassium needs must be verified with blood test.
- adrenal support—(where indicated) see Chapter 6.
- liver support—(where indicated) see Chapter 5

   (c)
- proteolytic enzymes (combined in one product)—to reduce inflammation and reduce pain and swelling (see Chapter 8).

   (d)
- Arginase—an enzyme necessary for the breakdown of argenine (a byproduct of protein metabolism which can build up in the kidneys). High arginine in the kidneys can create gout.

Individual requirements can vary, so consult your health professional. Work with your health professional to monitor results.

13. Herbs beneficial for gout: comfrey, parsley, alfalfa and ginger

14. Raw juices beneficial for gout: red sour cherries, black cherries, pineapple, potato, celery, carrot, dark greens and beets.

"Just as we would perish without food and water, we will perish once our bodies are deprived of the movement necessary to maintain our vital physiological systems."

—Pete Egoscue
Anatomical Functionalist

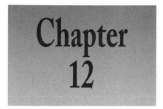

Chapter 12

Exercise & Arthritis

If you have arthritis, and as long as your physician feels your cartilage will not be damaged, you should be able to exercise. Well-conditioned and developed muscles act to absorb the shock that joints experience. Also, experts believe exercise enhances the release of the synovial fluid that bathes and nourishes cartilage. Regular aerobic exercise (such as walking, running and low-impact dancing) will help increase your flexibility, endurance and strength, as well as, aid in weight loss when needed. Gentle exercise, individually designed for you, will help preserve the mobility of arthritic joints. Your physician, along with an athletic trainer, exercise physiologist or physical therapist, can advise you as to what exercise best suits you, tailor it to your individual needs and enjoyment and offer motivation.

The following 12 steps are exercise and arthritis recommendations from Dr. Thomas K. Jamieson, an osteopathic physician specializing in family practice and sports medicine and owner of the Jamieson Total Health Care Center in Lansing, Michigan:

1. Stretch and warm up thoroughly before exercise. Cool down properly after exercise. Warm muscles and joints are more flexible and less apt to be strained or pulled.

2. During the day, use correct posture at rest, while sitting, standing and at play—avoid slouching.

3. Strive to maintain correct body weight. Obesity creates more stress and strain on weight-bearing joints (knees, hips and ankles), which can contribute to or cause osteoarthritis. According to research, losing even ten pounds may reduce your risk of osteoarthritis in the knees by 50 percent.

4. One of the least stressful exercises for your joints is walking or running on a rebounder (mini-trampoline) or treadmill. Use hand rails for balance and support, if needed. Both are beneficial for the lymphatic and circulatory systems and, like all exercise, can create a positive outlook and sense of well being.

   (a) When walking, wear appropriate shoes and comfortable clothing.

   (b) Start with a short time and distance and work up to longer increments. Example: 5 minutes the first week and then build up by adding 5 minutes each week, eventually walking 20 minutes to 30 minutes per day.

5. Swimming or warm-water exercise programs are ideal for joints and allow greater mobility for those suffering from acute and chronic symptoms of arthritis.

6. In cold weather, be sure to keep your joints warm with proper clothing and accessories (knee and feet socks, for example).

7. Rest, as needed. When injured or tired, your muscles are less able to help your joints and bones.

8. Heat relief. A warm bath or heating pad applied before exercise will help relax muscles and improve blood flow to both muscles and joints. Proper heat application can give relief from pain and swelling, thus making it easier to exercise.

Action creates "feel good" hormones.

Regular exercise releases "feel good" hormones called endorphins throughout your body which help to reduce pain and lifts your spirits. You feel actively involved in your health, in more control and develop improved self-esteem.

---

9. Never exercise when you have acute inflammation or injured joints without consulting your physician or physical therapist.

10. Individualized weight-training programs build strength and improve flexibility and endurance, while improving muscle balance and structural support.

11. Supervised exercise programs help ensure proper techniques and motivation, and alleviate any apprehension about exercise. Consider water exercise programs, Tai Chi, or yoga classes. Check with your local YMCA, athletic club and Arthritis Foundation office for specialized exercise programs for arthritis in your area.

12. Find an exercise and activity you enjoy or create enjoyment for it. If it's fun, you'll be more apt to stick with it and will consistently build strong bones, ligaments and muscles.

Exercise may not always relieve the pain from arthritis which is due to bone migration into soft tissue, stretched ligaments or the disease's effect on the subchondral bone (the bone under the cartilage). Yet, proper exercise can help reduce

> Moving a joint through its complete range of motion, then gently pushing it a little beyond that range, will improve flexibility and help reduce the pain.

pain from arthritis in many individuals. This relief may be from the stretching of contracted tissues, weak muscles getting stronger or from the release of natural pain controllers, called endorphins, from the brain.

Keep in mind that exercise is beneficial for arthritis mainly because it helps keep muscles and joints working as best they

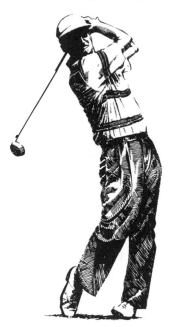

can, which then allows your whole body better support and function. Exercise prevents muscle atrophy and helps maintain and build muscle strength and range of motion. So exercise is certainly worth the effort when done properly.

Immobility has been shown to encourage arthritic changes in the joints. Immobility (lack of or even improper movement of joints) may deprive the joints of oxygen and a series of immune system steps may be set in motion. White blood cells may attack joint tissue, slowly destroying cartilage, ligaments, tendons and progressively making arthritis worse.

Find exercise you enjoy and make time for play and fun. You have a renewed sense of energy and empowerment.

"The causal chain that leads to arthritis may, indeed, begin with an environment that restricts movement

... the joint that doesn't move in a functional way and in sufficient amount, becomes one that cannot move at all, further grading the immune system," states Pete Egosure, expert in anatomical function.[30]

Pain Signals and Injury Prevention

1. Some extra pain and soreness should be expected on the first and second days of exercise and while performing the exercise. You should be safely able to continue your program.
2. Consult your physician (or physical therapist) if pain lasts more than two hours after exercise **or** of there is increased pain in a joint 24 hours after exercise. You should decrease the amount of exercise.
3. Your physician and/or physical therapist should inform you as to how much discomfort or pain is safe to experience and how much pain is a warning to reduce or stop exercise.
4. When experiencing pain, stop and rest.
5. Increase exercise gradually, to prevent injury.

Injury Care

If an injury has occurred:

1. Remember R.I.C.I.:

   - R = REST

   - I = ICE. Swelling can be reduced in the injured area with **ice**. Ice is always safe to use with an injury.

"Physical therapists tailor individual exercise and rehabilitation programs for each patient using a variety of modalities to increase strength, mobility and function of muscles and joints, while helping to relieve pain. Some of the most beneficial exercise programs for arthritis use pool therapy."— Teresa Jamieson, Physical Therapist, Lansing, Michigan

Acute injury (sprained ankle/pulled muscle): Ice 20 minutes every three to four hours, for 48 hours after the injury.

Do not apply ice directly to skin.

- C = COMPRESSION. Wrap the injured area with an ace bandage to prevent the swelling from migrating to other parts of the limb.

- E = ELEVATE injured area between icings. This retards swelling by reducing blood flow.

> Individuals with osteoarthritis, aged 40 to 89, volunteered for a study where they walked three times per week for 30 minutes and participated in a light stretching and strengthening program. After 8 weeks, the walkers demonstrated an average 15% increase in walking capacity and *no* increase in arthritis symptoms.
>
> Study done by Hospital for Special Surgery in New York City, 1992.

2. Heat should not be applied to an injury unless approved by your physician, athletic trainer or physical therapist. Heat may cause extreme swelling and create the need for prolonged rehabilitation.

3. If pain persists after two days and icing, compression and reduction or discontinuance of exercise have not worked, consult your physician.

4. If numbness or tingling sensations are present, it may indicate a serious injury—consult your physician.

Stretching Exercises

Stretching is a form of exercise that almost everyone with arthritis can do. Stretching will improve your flexibility, help your joints move in their proper range of motion, increase your circulation and energy and help relax your mind.

1. Use fluid movements as you stretch. Do not bounce or jerk.

2. Relax and breathe while stretching. Picture in your mind calm and soothing images (for example, think about floating in the sun on a raft). Breathe! Proper breathing helps reduce pain and allows more relaxation and fluid movement.

3. Do not strain. Stretch to the point of slight tension **before** developing pain.

4. Go to your limit of the stretch and hold. You may hold for 10 to 15 seconds until you are more relaxed. Gently push a little beyond the "limit" of the stretch to improve flexibility.

5. Concentrate on the area you are stretching (your shoulders, back or arms) and feel them losing their stiffness and tension.

6. You should work on a total body stretching program, progressing to the specific areas of your arthritis pain.

EXAMPLES OF STRETCHING EXERCISES:

1. UPPER BODY

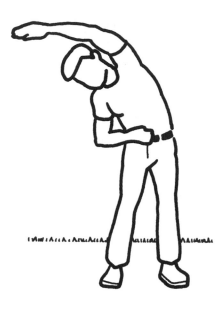

Side-Bending Stretch

With right hand pushing gently on right hip, reach with left arm. Repeat with opposite arm.

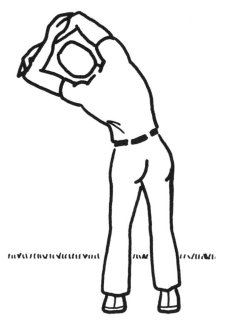

Cross-Arm Stretch

Cross your wrists and clasp your hands together as you reach your arms overhead. Keep reaching upward for several seconds.

1. UPPER BODY (continued)

Shoulder Stretch

With your right hand holding your left arm parallel to the floor, gently pull your left elbow across your chest toward your right shoulder and hold. Repeat with opposite shoulder.

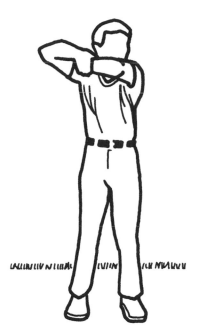

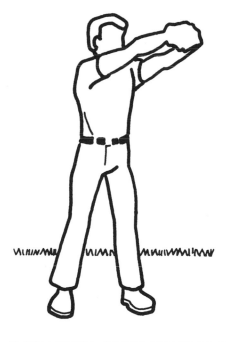

Front Arm Stretch

Stretch with both arms parallel to the floor, reach forward and clasp hands in front of you and hold. Now turn your clasped palms outward as you reach and stretch.

2. BACK AND TRUNK

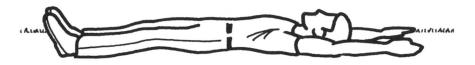

Elongation Stretch

Lie on floor with arms and legs extended to stretch entire body. Keep your lower back pressed to the floor throughout stretch.

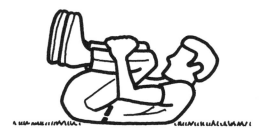

Tuck Stretch

Lie on back and slide feet slowly along floor while bringing knees toward your chest. At the same time, lift your head and shoulders off the floor while tucking in. Keep chin tucked toward your chest. Hold for 10 to 15 seconds. Then return to original position. Repeat three times.

3. LOWER BODY

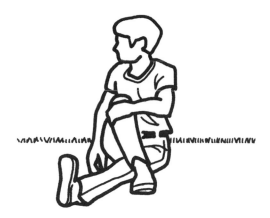

Hip Twister Stretch

Keeping your hips pressed down, gently pull your right knee toward your chest. Repeat with opposite knee

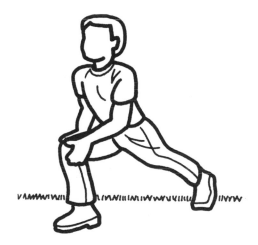

Standing Calf Stretch

Push against the wall as you keep the back heel pressed down. This stretches the calf of the rear leg. As your flexibility improves, push the rear heel further away from the wall. Repeat with opposite leg.

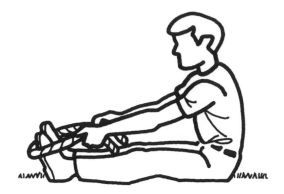

Sitting Calf Stretch

First, wrap a towel gently around the balls of your feet. With knees relaxed, pull the towel toward you.

Kneeling Stretch

With back knee on floor, move your front leg until your knee is directly over your ankle. Press your hips downward, gently. Repeat with opposite leg.

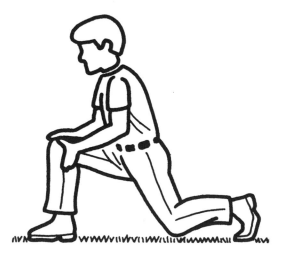

A comprehensive stretching and exercise program designed to balance the musculoskeletal system and improve function and healing is outlined in the book, *The Egoscue Method of Health Through Motion* created by anatomical functionalist, Pete Egoscue (Please see Appendix II). Dr. Jamieson, of the Jamieson Total Health Care Center, has used this program in his office for over three years with tremendous benefits for his patients.

NOTES

30. Egoscue, Pete, *The Egoscue Method of Health Through Motion*, Harper Collins, 1992, page 180.

"Manipulative therapy helps maintain the structural and functional integrity of the musculoskeletal system."

—The role of osteopathic and chiropractic manipulative therapy

Manipulative Therapy—Joint Movement for Healing

Manipulative therapy can help the joints become more mobile and prevent arthritic progression. Osteopathic and chiropractic manipulation or "mobilization" help to "free" the joint, allowing it to function as it was designed. Both osteopathic and chiropractic manipulative therapy are concerned with maintaining the structural and functional integrity of the musculoskeletal system.

Usually, the last thing you feel like doing when you have inflammation and joint pain is movement or activity of any kind. Yet, the **proper movement** of your joints is just the medicine they need—especially in arthritis. A joint is designed to perform in its proper range of movement, and inactivity may actually lead to a progression of arthritis.

Recent research has supported the idea that immobilization (bed rest, inactivity) can actually cause arthritis and also delay healing. After a 15-year study at the Institute of Occupational Health in Helsinki, Finland, T. Videman and co-researchers concluded that "immobilization, for whatever reason, is one of the pathogenic factors in musculoskeletal degeneration."[31]

Brock Walker, D.C., appointed to the American Back Society, and Secretary of the Executive Committee on Manipulative Medicine,

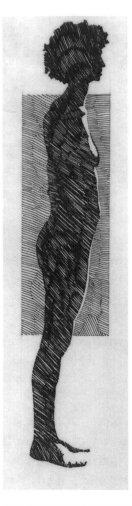

> Manipulative therapy can help ensure proper body alignment and improve muscle and joint function.

explains that if a joint is immobilized (either by injury, irritation or inflammation), the brain tells your muscles around that area to go into spasm to protect that joint. Spasms create pain and can lead to further immobilization and arthritic progression in the joint (fibrous tissue with calcium deposits, etc.).

To correct structural problems, a doctor skilled in manipulative therapy will use

꙾

Improper body alignment, poor muscle tone and bad pasture will aggravate arthritis pain and can contribute to the progression of the disease.

direct pressure or move specific muscles, bones and joints. The adjustments improve nerve function and improve blood flow to various areas of the body. Manipulative therapy balances posture and improves mobility, encouraging the body's natural ability to heal itself.

Proper manipulative therapy helps you maintain movement of the joints in their correct range, relieves pain and prevents further injury or degeneration. Thomas K. Jamieson, D.O., states that patients will respond best to manipulation when they practice good nutrition and stretch and exercise regularly. Avoiding caffeine and alcohol seems to have a positive effect on reducing inflammation, whether it be inflammation from arthritis or improper body alignment. Manipulative therapy helps support the whole bio-mechanical system by improving the health of the nervous system, organs and tissues.

NOTES

31. Videman, T., "Experimental Models of Osteoarthritis: The Role of Immobilization." *Clinical Biomechanics Magazine*, 1987 (2:223–229).

"The first secret you should know about perfect health is that you have to choose it. You can only be as healthy as you think it is possible to be."

—Maharishi Ayurveda

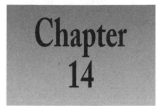

Chapter 14

Acupuncture and Arthritis

Acupuncture, a 5,000-year-old healing practice originating in China, is gaining acceptance in the United States as a respectable, noninvasive healing treatment. More and more physicians are recommending acupuncture to their patients as part of their treatment for asthma, allergies, back pain and a variety of other health problems. Acupuncture can be beneficial in arthritis for reduction of pain, and plays a role in holistic treatment since it is used to help re-establish stressed or imbalanced organ systems.

Supporting the belief that good health depends on the entire body being in balance, acupuncture treatment involves stimulation of the energy within the body. Small (virtually painless) needles are inserted into specific points on the skin's surface. These points relate to the flow of energy in pathways called meridians. According to theory, by stimulating the flow of energy through the meridians, healing can take place in stressed organs and systems.

Renée Hubbs, certified acupuncturist and practitioner at the Meridian Health and Wellness Center in East Lansing, Michigan, explains the benefits:

> "Acupuncture inhibits the pain signals sent to the brain through a mild, fairly painless stimulation by closing the gates of the pain-signaling system. This prevents the sensations of pain from traveling through the spinal cord to the brain. As the area is released, the muscle fibers elongate and relax, enabling the blood to flow smoothly, and toxins are released and eliminated. Increased circulation also brings more oxygen and other nutrients to the affected areas, which increases the body's resistance to illness and promotes a longer, healthier, more vital life. When the blood and bio-electrical energy circulate properly, we have a greater sense of harmony, health and well-being."

Prior to the acupuncture treatment itself, the acupuncturist will assess the state of the meridians by feeling different pulse variations and by looking at the tongue's shape, color and surface. These assessments reveal which meridians need to be balanced. For example: If the energy pathway corresponding to the liver is underactive, the acupuncturist will stimulate this area with acupuncture to bring it up to normal.

Acupuncture treatment can involve fine-tipped acupuncture needles, electro-acupuncture or heat application (thermal therapy) using moxibustion (heat herbal treatment), or a combination of these techniques.

In conjunction with the above techniques, Chinese herbal remedies would be suggested by an acupuncurist. These herbal remedies are prescribed according to an individual's constitutional needs, based on their excess or deficient readings of their pulse and tongue diagnosis.

It is important to note that patients must be seen by a qualified acupuncturist to have their individual concerns supported. Over-the-counter suggestions in a store do not address each person's unique constitutional needs, may even create an imbalance (an excess or deficiency), or be of no benefit to the condition. Herbal remedies are specific to individual needs.

Bruce H. Pomeranz, M.D., a neurologist at the University of Toronto, has found evidence that acupuncture releases endorphins, which are hormones involved with pain relief and a sense of well-being. The Chinese and other Eastern cultures have successfully used acupuncture for pain control and anesthesia for many years, and the Western world is recognizing its benefits more and more.

Deborah Lincoln, R.N., board-certified acupuncturist, president of the Michigan Acupuncture Coalition and owner of Meridian Health and Wellness Center in East Lansing, Michigan, confirms the complementary benefits of acupuncture with Western medicine, and states that "acupuncture is a complete medical system and, due to its proven effectiveness, has been embraced throughout the world."

A qualified acupuncturist can be found through a physician's referral or phone directory. Look for a nationally certified acupuncturist—ideally one with many years of experience.

> "... acupuncture inhibits the pain signals sent to the brain ..."

"The way to health is to have an aromatic bath and scented massage every day."

—Hippocrates
The father of modern medicine

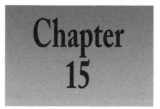

Healing Touch • Massage and Aromatherapy

Consider how our body responds to touch when we rub a sore leg muscle or press our temple when our head pounds from a headache. Both are sometimes automatic actions we do to ourselves when our body signals it is in pain. We are instinctively practicing massage and acupressure. Yes, sometimes without realizing it, we give our body just what it needs to feel better.

Massage is excellent therapy for the body and has been recognized for thousands of years as a healing tool. In ancient Greece and Rome, massage was a main form of healing and pain relief. In the beginning of the nineteenth century, Swedish massage was developed by Per Henrik Long and the first school of massage was started in Sweden in 1813.

For thousands of years, the Oriental world has used various forms of acupressure massage—called Shiatsu—and even reflexology (pressure applied by the thumbs or fingers to reflex points on the hands and feet). Records show reflexology was even practiced in ancient Egypt.

The Western World has finally recognized that massage (therapeutic, Shiatsu and reflexology) is beneficial in health care. The various forms of massage can stimulate healing and cleansing in the body and thus be beneficial for the prevention and treatment of arthritis pain. Therapeutic massage involves a systematic method of kneading, pressing and stroking the muscles, tendons and ligaments. By relaxing these soft tissues, pain from tension and stress, aggravated by stiffness due to arthritis, can be reduced. Not only is massage relaxing, but therapeutically, it can improve blood circulation and lymphatic flow.

Shiatsu. A Japanese form of body work, Shiatsu is more like a form of physical therapy in that it encompasses stimulation of the acupressure points throughout the body that correspond to the meridian pathways that relate to energy flow in the body. Indirectly, Shiatsu affects the muscles, circulation, and lymphatics. More directly, it helps energize the body and relieve blocked energy pathways to the organ systems by the stimulation of pressure points.

Reflexology. Based in part on similar beliefs and principles of acupressure, reflexology involves the application of pressure to the reflex points on the feet or hands. These reflex points are the points of termination for the energy channels flowing throughout the body. With disease or illness, such as arthritis, organ systems may become weak or sick due to the blockage of the energy channels.

Aromatherapy. A traditional therapy dating back to 1580 BC with Egyptians using the aromatic properties produced from many different herbal plants. Hippocrates, the father of modern medicine, said, "The way to health is to have an aromatic bath and scented massage every day."

Aromatherapy can be helpful to relieve pain and is an effective muscle relaxant when used in a massage oil, in compresses or with bath therapy. Often times, the joint areas are too inflamed, painful or swollen to massage with aromatic oils, so baths or compresses are excellent natural treatments.

Generally, aromatherapy oils are mixed in a carrier oil before you apply them to the skin for a compress or massage treatment. The typical carrier oils used are almond kernel, apricot kernel, peach kernel or grapeseed oil. You can use any cold-pressed vegetable oil, also. Oils turn rancid with oxidation, so store in dark glass bottles which are tightly closed.

Therapeutic massage, acupressure, reflexology and aromatherapy may be incorporated in one massage treatment or can be used separately as unique applications on their own. Massage stimulates the circulation, nervous system, and lymphatics, and aids digestion and elimination. In other words, it can benefit

Aromatherapy Oils Beneficial to Arthritis

Basil	•Lemon
Benzoin resin*	•Marjoram*
Black pepper*	Myrrh
Cedarwood	•Pine
•Chamomile*	•Rosemary*
Clove*	Tyme
•Coriander*	•Vetiver
Elemi	•Juniper
•Eucalyptus*	•Ginger*
Fennel	Frankincense*
Helichrysum	

*Aromatherpy oils marked by a • or * are those most commonly used.*

• Add 1 to 2 drops of 1 to 3 of these oils to a carrier oil to use for aromatheapy massage treatment.

* Blend 2 to 3 drops of 2 to 3 of these oils and add to both water or use as a compress.

the whole body chemistry which then supports arthritis relief or prevention.

Massage is a healthy, noninvasive way to help your body chemistry, but remember these points:

1. Look for a licensed massage therapist. You can get excellent referrals from your city's area massage association, the American Massage Association, and physicians.

2. Talk with your physician concern ing any precautions your massage therapist should be aware of with your arthritis and health history. Massage should not be done over an acute inflammatory condition or directly on the joint itself. Massage the soft tissue around the joint.

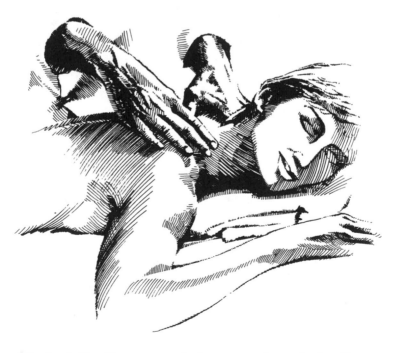

Manipulative therapy can help ensure proper body alignment and improve muscle and joint function.

3. Communicate with your massage therapist before and during your massage treatment, so she or he is aware of any unusual discomfort or pain you might be experiencing.

4. Relax, enjoy, and allow your body to experience the healing within itself

Soothing Bath

Aromatherapy bath to ease arthritis pain. Try soaking in a warm bath with a few drops of juniper oil added

Aromatherapy massage recipe

Blend 5 drops of eucalyptus oil with 10 drops each of frankincense and rosemary. Add to carrier oil.

*"There is consciousness in
every single cell of the body."*

—Deepak Chopra, M.D.

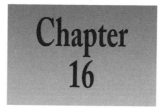

Chapter 16

The Mind-Body Connection

How would you feel if you put a smile on your face right now? A big, warm smile and a twinkle in your eyes makes you feel better, doesn't it? Even if you were frustrated about your painful joints, it would be hard to have the same level of frustration or pain if you put a big smile on your face.

Now try this: Close your eyes and imagine you are in your favorite place—perhaps on a warm, sunny beach. As you vividly create this image and use all your favorite colors and sounds and emotions, can't you feel the muscles in your body relax?

Yes, there is a strong interaction or link between the mind and the body. They each influence one another. One of the quickest ways to link the mind and body is through correct breathing, such as with **deep diaphragmatic breathing exercises, yoga,** or **transcendental meditation**. Breathing deeply relaxes the mind. Under stress, we tend to take shallow breaths. When we are in physical pain, we also tend to tense up and breathe shallowly. Breathing deeply is one way to induce relaxation of mind and body. Harvard Medical School professor Herbert Benson, M.D., did a 20-year clinical study and found strong support for the ability of relaxation to reduce the symptoms of stress and stress-related illness.

Breathing patterns are one way to relax the body and help reduce stress and physical pain. Another way to help link the mind and body is through **visualization**, **imagery**, **hypnosis**, or **biofeedback** training. Each has its own unique application. It is not the focus of this book to explain each in detail, but instead, to remind ourselves of the tremendous impact the mind has on our well-being.

In his best-selling book, *Love, Medicine and Miracles*, Bernie Siegel, M.D., relates his own personal, as well as his patients' experiences with the impact that attitudes, beliefs and goals have on the healing process and prognosis of disease. Working with cancer patients, Dr. Siegel found that those patients who had a sense of "purpose in life"—something to live for and feelings that they had choices with their health care and life—had better recovery from illness or lived longer.[32]

Norman Cousins, author of *Anatomy of an Illness*, states, ". . . the most important knowledge in medicine to be learned or taught is in the way the human mind and body can summon innermost resources to meet extraordinary challenges."[33] **Laughter, humor, love, comfort** and all the other **positive emotions** human beings are capable of expressing can be amazing healers. We just need to express and be open to these basic nutrients for the mind. Feeding the mind positive thoughts and images may not "cure" arthritis or any disease, but it is vital to the health of the whole person, and assists the body in healing.

Having the proper mental attitude and faith is not meant to be a cure-all or "quick fix." There are really no quick solutions when it comes to arthritis or any disease. The body takes time to heal, and there are many choices we can make to help this process.

However, even when you have choices, you don't always take the necessary actions to get results. Sometimes you're not motivated to change your eating habits, you're bored with exercise or afraid to seek medical advice about arthritis—fearing the unknown. All these mindsets keep you from behaviors that could give you healthy results. You get "stuck" in a mindset, and feel handicapped, and then poor habits and attitudes can lead to unhealthy outcomes.

One of the most successful and exciting ways we can learn to break out of these unproductive habits and make change is a technology called **Neuro-Associative Conditioning Techniques** (NAC^{TM}),[34] developed and taught by Anthony Robbins. NAC^{TM} is based, in part, on **Neuro-Linguistic Programming (NLP)**, a science of personal development studying human excellence as well as other behavioral sciences which influence change and personal growth. Psychologists, teachers, health professionals and business people nationwide are recognizing these techniques as a powerful breakthrough in personal development. In his best-selling book, Unlimited Power, Anthony Robbins explains how we can change our states and outcomes in life **by changing our focus** (internal representations) and **changing our physiology** (body language).:

He states, "If you change your physiology—that is, your posture, your breathing patterns, your muscle tension, your tonality—you instantly change your internal representations and your state." It is a cybernetic loop—the mind influences the body and the body influences the mind.

Hypnotherapy is rapidly gaining the recognition it has long deserved for its benefits in pain control and mind/body healing. "Health professionals are recognizing hypnotherapy's effect in

Chronic and acute pain can cause frustration, stress and even depression. Mind-body tools can empower you and break the cycle of pain and feelings of helplessness.

Learn to manage and cope with arthritis pain by learning and practicing effective mind-body techniques such as
- ~biofeedback
- ~progressive relaxation
- ~meditation
- ~guided imagery
- ~hypnotherapy

changing the pain threshold to the degree, in some cases, that it may be even more effective than narcotic agents for relief or elimination of pain. Hypnosis can help empower us to take charge of our health through the power of the mind," according to Robert Ranger, clinical hypnotherapist and founding director of the Institute of Transformational Hypnotherapy in Michigan.

Hypnosis is a naturally occurring state of the mind which allows us to move with our own volition to a natural state of focused concentration in which we can use more of our subconscious mind. Positive suggestions for healing and personal development enable the subconscious mind to assist the body's innate ability to heal.

A certified hypnotherapist is a coach who is skilled at teaching safe, effective and comfortable strategies (including self-hypnosis) to help you use your mind and improve your health and manage pain. Your hypnotherapist will use and teach you how to reach this state of focused concentration by using deep relaxation and visualization techniques.

Progressive relaxation, visualization, and guided imagery are some of the methods used in hypnosis as well as in meditation and biofeedback. Please refer to Appendix III in this book for additional resources to learn more about these methods. When we learn and regularly practice these tools for managing our thoughts and body functions, they can help to relieve the perception of pain and can even alter the body's chemistry, which creates pain. Seek the support, wisdom, expertise of professionals in your area who offer either individual sessions or workshops and classes in mind/body principles.

NOTES

32. Siegel, Bernie, M.D., *Love, Medicine and Miracles*, New York: Harper and Row, 1986.

33. Cousins, Norman, *Anatomy of an Illness*, New York: Norton and Company, 1979.

34. Robbins, Anthony, *Unlimited Power*, New York: Simon and Schuster, 1986 (p. 141).

"Let food be your medicine"

—Hippocrates

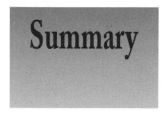

Summary

Surgery (such as joint replacement or reconstruction) may not be necessary if you start good health habits early to slow or alleviate the progression of arthritis. Seek medical and health advice early when the swelling and discomfort first starts.

Remember these early warning signs of arthritis:

1. pain in joints

2. stiffness upon rising, persisting for two or three hours

3. inflammation, pink and red joints

4. joints warm to the touch

5. swollen joints

The above symptoms, especially when the cause is left untreated, can lead to destruction of the joint. At this stage, surgery may be necessary. It is important to have a correct diagnosis so the proper treatment can be initiated.

Arthritis need not be a crippling and painful disease. Seek advice early and take part in your health care.

Prevention and natural therapy can work alongside traditional medical care. *Breakthroughs in Natural Healing* require, first—breaking through those old beliefs and habits that cause barriers to optimum health. Choose to take action and take control of your health and well-being.

Take care of your body and it will take care of you!

Glossary of Terms

allergens—substances that induce an allergic reaction. (Allergens are thought to be linked to the body's overload of toxins where an "overwhelmed" body overreacts to things that may otherwise be harmless.)

amoeba (amoebic)—a single-cell protozoan animal form. The amoeba species entamoeba is parasitic to humans.

ankylosing spondylitis—an inflammatory condition which causes immobility of the vertebrae.

antibodies—specialized proteins produced in the body in response to substances such as infectious agents or foreign matter.

arthritis—inflammation of one or more joints; arth means joint; itis means inflammation.

auto-antibodies—abnormal antibodies directed against parts of a person's own body rather than against invading antigens.

auto-immune disease—a condition in which the body has developed a sensitivity to some of its own tissue.

basophil—a special type of white blood cell that digests and renders toxins harmless.

bone—the hard tissue which forms the skeleton or framework of the body; bone is composed of calcium and other minerals and elastic tissues.

bursae (bursa = singular)—small pockets or sac-like cavities in or near the joints which contain the synovial fluids that protect the movable joints from friction.

bursitis—inflammation of the bursae (or bursa).

cartilage—the cartilage protects movable joints against friction and absorbs shock. There are 3 types of cartilage: hyaline, fibro cartilage and elastic cartilage. Unlike bone tissue. cartilage has no blood vessels.

chondral—pertaining to cartilage; **chondro**—a prefix meaning cartilage.

collagen—the main structural protein of connective tissue.

endorphins—naturally occurring compounds with pain-relieving properties.

eosinophil—a white blood cell (granular leukocyte) that digests harmful micro-organisims.

gout—a disease which there is a upset in the metabolism of uric acid causing joint inflammation and pain.

heberden's nodes—enlargements of the fingers or toes at the last joint (closest to the nail); found in osteoarthritis.

IgG4—an antibody; a subclass of the whole IgE molecule associated with a delayed food reaction, when elevated.

IgE—an antibody in the blood associated with immediate allergic response, when elevated.

immune (immunity)—protected against disease; able to resist diseases.

joint—a place where two or more bones or cartilage come together (example: hip and shoulder joints).

ligaments—fibrous bands that hold bones together in the region of a joint.

lymphocytes—white blood cells that lack granulocytes, which are found in blood and lymphoid tissue.

[T-lymphocytes—a type of white blood cell made in the bone marrow programmed to detect and destroy enemy substances.]

[B-lymphocytes—a type of white blood cell that produces antibodies that neutralize and erase a wide range of allergy-causing invaders.]

mast cells—specialized cells found in tissues. These granule-containing cells release chemicals that create arthritis symptoms.

monocytes—a large type of white blood cell that scavenges and destroys harmful bacteria and other foreign matter.

muscle—the tissue responsible for body movement; the body has over 600 different muscles.

node—enlargement of the fingers or toes at the joint, caused by bony growths (In osteoarthritis the enlargements are at the last joint closest to the nails and are called Heberden's nodes).

osteoarthritis—a degenerative joint disease caused by a combination of irritation, injury to the joints, normal wear and tear, and "aging."

phagocyte—a type of white blood cell that absorbs or engulfs a foreign substance.

rheumatoid arthritis—pain, swelling, and deformity of the joints. Although the cause(s) is unknown, experts believe it is an auto-immune disease.

Rh Factor—a substance found in the red blood cells.

SED rate (sedimentation rate or Erythrocyte Sedimentation Rate)—a blood test used by physicians to diagnose inflammatory diseases, including rheumatoid arthritis. A measure of how fast erythrocytes (red blood cells) fall to the bottom of a tube filled with whole blood. If elevated, it can be an indication of inflammation.

subchondrial bone—pertaining to bone below or under cartilage.

spondyle—vertebrae

spondylitis—inflammation of the spine.

spur—a pointed outgrowth on the bone.

synovial fluid—clear, lubricating fluid secreted by the synovial membrane of the joint.

synovial membranes—membranes that serve as linings for joints and secrete synovial fluid.

synovitis—inflammation of the lining of the joint (synovial membrane).

synovium—the capsule that surrounds the joint and contains synovial fluid.

tendon—fibrous tissue that connects muscle to other tissue.

white blood cells—leukocytes or white corpuscles.

white blood count differential—a blood test which measures the separate white blood cell components: neutrophils, eosinophils, basophils, lymphocytes and monocytes.

Appendix I

Newsletters/Magazines

Alternative Medicine Digest. Future Medicine Pub., Inc., 1640 Tuburon Blvd. #2, Tuburon, CA 94920 (415) 435-1779.

Health Alert Newsletter, P.O. Box 22620, Carmel, CA 93922-2620 (408) 372-2103. Published by Dr. Bruce West.

Nutrition Action Newsletter, Center for Science in the Public Interest, Ste. 300, 1875 Connecticut Ave., N.W., Washington, D.C. 20009-5728

The Journal of the National Academy of Research Biochemists, 750 Rancho Circle, Fullerton, CA 92635 (714) 992-0616

Laboratories

These laboratories offer trace mineral/hair analysis, Comprehensive Stool and Digestive Analysis, IgG4 allergy tests, adrenal stress tests and other specialized lab tests)

Meridian Valley Lab, 515 West Harrison St.
Ste. 9, Kent, WA 98032 (800) 234-6825 ext. 156

Metametrix Laboratory
5000 Peachtree Industrial Blvd., Ste 110
Norcross, GA 30071
(800) 221-4640

Great Smokies Lab
18A Regent Park Blvd.
Ashville, NC 28816
(800) 522-4762

Diagnos-Techs, Inc.
P.O. Box 58948
Seattle, WA 98138
(206) 251-0596

Consult with physicians in your area who are familiar with these lab tests to evaluate digestive abnormalities (intestinal dysbiosis), food allergy screening, adrenal stress tests and mineral analysis. The lab work must be ordered by a physician.

Where to get organic produce:

—Visit food co-operatives and health-food markets in your area

Or contact these resources:

—Whole Food Direct
  800-721-1400

—Americans for Safe Food
  1875 Connecticut Avenue, N.W.
  Washington, DC 2009-5728
  202-332-9110

Source for Celtic Sea Salt:

—Grain and Salt Society
  800-867-7258

or check your local food co-operative or health food market

Where to find kitchen appliances for juicing foods:

Check your local food co-operative or health food store or contact:

—Vita Mix® Corp.
  8615 Usher Rd.
  Cleveland, OH 44138
  800-848-2649

—Champion™, Acme™ or other juicers:

  Acme Equipment
  1024 Concert Ave.
  Springhills, FL 34609
  800-882-0157

Appendix II

Additional Reading and Resources

Airola, Paavo, Ph.D., N.D. *How to Get Well*. Phoenix: Health Plus Pub., 1974.

Anderson, Bob. *Stretching*. P.O. Box 2734, Fullerton, CA 92633, 1975.

Baker, Elizabeth, and Dr. Elton. *The Uncook Book*. Sagauche, CO: Drelwood Pub., 1983.

Budwig, Johanna, Ph.D. *Flax Oil as a True Aid Against Arthritis, Heart Infarction, Cancer and Other Diseases*. Vancouver, BC: Apple Pub., 1993.

Chang, Dr. Stephen Thomas. *The Complete Book of Acupuncture*. Berkeley, CA: Celestial Arts, 1976.

Chopra, Deepak, M.D. *Perfect Health*. New York: Harmony Books, 199. The Chopra Center for Wellbeing, LaJolla, CA

Czaplicki, Roman. *Acupuncture, 5000 Years of Healing Art*. Warren, MI: 1974.

Deal, Sheldon C., D.C. *New Life Through Nutrition*. Tucson: New Life Pub., 1974.

Egoscue, Pete. *The Egoscue Method of Health Through Motion*. New York: Harper Collins Pub., 1992.

Fredericks, Carlton. *Program for Living Longer*. New York: Simon and Schuster, 1983.

Galland, Leo., M.D. *Superimmunity for Kids*. New York: Copestone Press, 1988.

Hill, Ann, editor. *A Visual Encyclopedia of Unconventional Medicine, A Health Manual for the Whole Person.* New York: Crown Pub., 1979.

Jarvis, D.C., M.D. *Arthritis and Folk Medicine.* New York: Holt, Rinehart and Winston, 1958.

Jenson, Dr. Bernard, and Anderson, Mark. *Empty Harvest.* Garden City, New York: Avery Pub., 1990.

Lidell, Lucinda. *The Book of Massage.* New York: Simon and Schuster, 1984.

Lockie, Andrew, M.D., and Geddes, Nicole, M.D. *The Complete Guide to Homeopathy.* New York:

Lopez, D.A., M.D.; Williams, R.M., M.D.; Ph.D.; M. Miehlke, M.D. *Enzymes The Fountain of Life.* Charleston, S.C.: Neville Press, 1994.

Mendelsohn, Robert S., M.D. *Confessions of a Medical Heretic.* Pickering, Ontario: Beaverbooks, 1979.

Mendleson, Robert S., M.D. *How to Raise a Healthy Child . . . in Spite of Your Doctor.* Chicago: Contemporary Books, Inc., 1984.

Mole, Peter. *Health Essential Acupuncture.* New York: Penguin USA, 1992.

Nitler, Dr. Alan H. *A New Breed of Doctor.* New York: Pyramid House, 1972

Oski, Frank A., M.D. *Don't Drink Your Milk.* New York: Mollica Press, Ltd., 1983.

Pfeiffer, Carl C., Ph.D. *Zinc and Other Micro-Nutrients.* New Canaan, CN: Keats Pub., 1978.

Price, Weston. *Nutrition and Physical Degeneration.* San Diego: Price-Pottenger Nutrition Federation, 1939.

Robbins, Anthony. *Unlimited Power.* New York: Simon and Schuster, 1986. Also available through Robbins Research International: Anthony Robbins Personal Power II, The Driving Force!—30-day Personal Power audio tapes. 800-445-8183.

Siegel, Bernie, M.D. *Love, Medicine and Miracles*. New York: Harper and Row Pub., 1986.

Ullman, Dana, M.P.H. and Stephen Cummings, M.D., *Everybody's Guide to Homeopathy*.

Wright, Johnathon V., M.D. *Wright's Book of Nutritional Therapy*. Emmaus, PA: Rodale Press, Inc., 1979.

Appendix III

Associations

—Arthritis Foundation
  P.O. Box 7669
  Atlanta, GA 30357-0669
  800-283-7800

—The Arthritis Hotline
  900-230-4800, ext. 7121

—National Chronic Pain Outreach Association
  7979 Old Georgetown Road, Ste. 100
  Bethesda, MD 20817
  301-652-4948

—American Pain Society
  5700 Old Orchard Road
  Skokie, IL 60077
  708-966-5595

—Osteopathic Medicine/Manipulative Therapy
  The American Osteopathic Association
  142 East Ontario Street
  Chicago, IL 60611
  313-280-5800

—International Chiropractors Association
  1110 North Glebe Road, Ste. 1000
  Arlington, VA 22201
  703-528-5000

—American Medical Association
  515 N. State St.
  Chicago, IL 60610
  312-464-5000

—American Association of Naturopathic Physicians
  2366 E. Lake Avenue
  Ste. 322
  Seattle, WA 98102
  206-323-7610

—American Association of Oriental Medicine
  433 Front Street
  Catasauga, PA 18032
  610-433-2448

—American Holistic Medical Association
  4101 Lake Bone Trail, Ste. 201
  Raleigh, NC 27607
  919-787-5146

—American Academy of Allergy and Immunology
  611 E. Wells Street
  Milwaukee, WI 53202
  800-822-2762

—Feingold Association of the United States
  U.S. Box 6550
  Alexandria, VA 22306
  703-768-3287
  Information on the effects of food and food additives on
  health, behavior and learning.

—Food Allergy Network
  4744 Holly Avenue
  Fairfax, VA 22030-5647
  703-691-3179

—American Physical Therapy Association
1111 Fairfax St.
Alexandria, VA 22314-1488
800-999-2782

—Biofeedback Certification Institute of America
10200 West 44th Avenue, Ste. 304
Wheat Ridge, CO 80033
303-420-2902

—American Society of Clinical Hypnotherapists
2250 E. Devon Save., Ste. 336
Des Plaines, IL 60018-4534
708-297-3317

—Milton Erickson Society for Psychotherapy and
Hypnotherapy
P.O. Box 1390
Madison Sq. Station
New York, NY 10159
212-628-0287

—Institute of Transformational Hypnotherapy
(Fully accredited training and hypnotherapy certification)
P.O. Box 1293
East Lansing, MI 48826
517-374-6156

—NLP Comprehensive Neuro-Linguistic
Programming Training
2897 Valmont Road
Boulder, CO 80302
800-233-1657

—Guided Imagery Therapy
Academy for Guided Imagery
P.O. Box 2070
Mill Valley, CA 94942
415-389-9324

—American Massage Therapy Association
  820 Davis St., Ste. 100
  Evanston, IL 60201
  708-864-0123

—The Chopra Center for Wellbeing
  Deepak Chopra, M.D.
  7630 Fay
  LaJolla, CA 92037
  619-551-7788

—National Association of Holistic Aromatherapy
  P.O. Box 17622
  Boulder, CO 80308-7622
  303-444-0533

Index

A

acidophilus, 42

adrenal, 63, 69, 74, 75, 83, 88, 89, 90, 91, 92, 93, 114, 122

alfalfa, 54, 55, 69, 82, 86, 122, 123

allergies, 37, 47, 48, 49, 50, 88, 89, 143

almonds, 37, 38, 49, 79, 80

amino acids, 35, 43, 48, 53, 54, 59, 63, 65, 70, 87, 99, 115

amylase, 41, 85, 104, 114

anti-inflammatory, 61, 62, 67, 69, 71, 74, 80, 84, 86, 88, 95, 96, 97, 98, 104, 114

anti-oxidant, 59, 72, 86, 95, 96, 97, 98, 99, 100, 104, 113

apple cider vinegar, 42

arnica, 94

auto-immune, 20, 45, 78, 95, 109

Ayurveda, 56, 142

B

bacteria, 39, 40, 42, 45, 111

basil, 149

beans, 34, 39, 73, 74, 79, 91, 99

beets, 42, 54, 55, 79, 82, 123

benzoin resin, 149

betaine, 42, 54, 56, 93

betaine hydrochloride, 41

bile, 42, 44, 54, 59

bioflavinoids, 75, 98

biotin, 73

black current seed oil, 78, 97, 114

black pepper, 149

boron, 63, 79, 112, 113

boswellia, 96

brewer's yeast, 69, 73, 79, 82, 83, 87, 88, 91, 120

bromelain, 41, 85, 96, 104, 114

bursa (bursae), 21

Bryonia, 94

C

caffeine, 91, 105, 116, 141

calcium, 35, 37, 40, 42, 43, 45, 54, 73, 76, 77, 78, 79, 81, 82, 87, 88, 91, 104, 105, 112, 140

capsaicin, 96

cartilage, 19, 20, 24, 33, 62, 65, 66, 67, 69, 71, 72, 75, 77, 98, 104, 125, 128

cat's claw, 97

cayenne, 96

cedarwood, 149

celery, 33, 75, 88, 91, 96, 97, 123

chamomile, 149

cherries, 88, 96, 121, 123

chili peppers, 96, 98

chlorophyll, 42, 69, 78, 81, 85, 86

chromium, 79

chondrocytes, 66

chondroitin sulfates, 62, 66, 67, 69, 70, 71, 72, 104, 114

cobalt, 79

collagen, 62, 65, 66, 74, 75

comfrey, 42, 123

Comprehensive Stool and Digestive Analysis (CSDA), 59, 111, 112

compresses, 149

connective tissue, 66, 74, 81, 82

copper, 72, 78, 80, 93, 112, 113

coriander, 149

curcumin, 97

Share *Arthritis Relief! Breakthroughs in Natural Healing* and a wealth of information for vibrant health with a family member or friend . . .

To obtain copies, visit your local bookstore or call 1-888-567-3363 or 1-888-KORDENE. (Also available in audiotape for your listening library.)

Send your check or money order to:
KORDENE PUBLICATIONS
4463 Copperhill Drive
Okemos, MI 48864

ISBN 1-890394-04-1

Send:____ at $ 14.95* each plus shipping/handling: $3.50 per book or audiotape (5 copies of more, $2.00 s/h per book)

Michigan residents add 6% sales tax per book
Outside the United States, Canadian price is $18.00 each, plus $5.00 s/h per book or audiotape.

Payment enclosed (check or money order) $_____
(Make checks payable to KORDENE PUBLICATIONS. Sorry, no credit cards accepted.)

Please print name _____

Address _____ Apt. #_____

City _____ State _____ Zip _____

SHIP TO: (if different from above)

Please print name _____

Address _____ Apt. #_____

City _____ State _____ Zip _____

*1998 Prices subject to change without notice.

_____